DIFFUSING ANGER

ANGER MANAGEMENT FOR PARENTS: MITIGATE TRIGGERS AND TAKE 3-STEP QUICK-RELEASE ACTION TO RAISE HAPPY, CONFIDENT CHILDREN

SASHA WOODLEY

© **Copyright 2023 Sasha Woodley - All rights reserved.**

The content contained within this book may not be reproduced, duplicated, or transmitted without direct written permission from the author or the publisher.

Under no circumstances will any blame or legal responsibility be held against the publisher, or author, for any damages, reparation, or monetary loss due to the information contained within this book, either directly or indirectly.

Legal Notice:

This book is copyright protected. It is only for personal use. You cannot amend, distribute, sell, use, quote or paraphrase any part, or the content within this book, without the consent of the author or publisher.

Disclaimer Notice:

Please note the information contained within this document is for educational and entertainment purposes only. All effort has been executed to present accurate, up-to-date, reliable, and complete information. No warranties of any kind are declared or implied. Readers acknowledge that the author is not engaged in the rendering of legal, financial, medical, or professional advice. The content within this book has been derived from various sources. Please consult a licensed professional before attempting any techniques outlined in this book.

By reading this document, the reader agrees that under no circumstances is the author responsible for any losses, direct or indirect, that are incurred as a result of the use of the information contained within this document, including, but not limited to, errors, omissions, or inaccuracies.

CONTENTS

Introduction	7
1. UNDERSTANDING YOUR ANGER	17
Uncontrolled Anger	21
Where Does Anger Come From?	24
Uncontrolled Anger May Damage Your Health	26
Psychological Effects of Anger	30
Positive Aspects of Anger	31
Parental Anger	32
2. WHAT MAKES YOU AN ANGRY PARENT? ALL ABOUT TRIGGERS	35
Managing Expectations	38
Anger's Triggers	40
Common Challenges for Short-Fused Parents	48
Controlling Your Temper as a Parent	50
Managing Your Triggers	53
3. LOVE YOURSELF—AND MITIGATE INVISIBLE TRIGGERS	55
Seeking Help	56
Who Are You Really?	60
Visualize a Positive Relationship With Your Child	63
Creating Some "Me" Time	63
Learn to Say "No"	64
Take Good Care of Yourself	66
Are You Feeding Your Anger?	71
Cultivating a Positive Mindset	74

How to Trick Your Brain Into Feeling Happy	76
Keys to Good Anger Management	79
Parents as Role Models	81

4. BECOMING A PEACEFUL PARENT — 85

Be Prepared: What to Expect From Your Kids	87
Five Stages of Human Development	88
Do Not Be an Emotional Enslaved Person	96
Parenting Imperfect	97
Put Yourself in Your Kid's Shoes	99
Why Do My Children Only Listen When I Yell?	101
Dealing With Sibling Rivalry	103
Coping With Tantrums and Meltdowns	106
What to Do When Your Child Is Angry: Hints and Tips	109

5. STAYING CALM WHEN YOUR CHILDREN PUSH YOUR BUTTONS — 117

Expressing Your Anger Constructively	118
Three-Step NPA Action For Instant Release	124
Other Ways to Deal With Anger Constructively	129
Meditation for Long-Term Anger Management	131

6. DIFFUSING PARENTAL ANGER — 139

A Useful Tip	140
Express Yourself in a Mindful Way	141
Communicate With Your Children	142
Take Action to Resolve the Triggers	144
Keep Your Trigger List Up to Date	144
Use Calming Herbs	147
Other Useful Supplements for Anger Management	152

7. THREE KEY INGREDIENTS TO RAISE
   WILLING, SELF-REGULATED
   CHILDREN   155
   Fostering a Good Relationship   155
   Allow Freedom of Expression   161
   Loving Unconditionally   165

   Conclusion   169
   References   173

INTRODUCTION

He was pouring his heart out on social media, hoping someone would listen: "I don't know why I'm always angry for no reason and explode without warning. Even trivial things trigger me, and I lash out, saying awful things I don't mean—and regret afterwards. My heart pounds really fast, and I can't control it. I literally get red tunnel vision. This happens to me almost every single day. I'm terrified that my rage is going to kill me."

If anger had a color palette, it would be in shades of red and purple, starting off with mauve for mild irritation or annoyance, escalating to red-hot outrage, and then deep violet-purple or even purple-black. Anger can be like a thunderstorm, starting with fluffy clouds and miniature storm cells, escalating into a battleship gray mass that blots out the sun, shot through with brilliant lightning bolts and the roar of thunderous shouting. The difference is that thunderstorms provide life-giving water and nitrogen, while the wild tempests of uncontrolled rage leave their victims hollow-eyed and exhausted, like hurricane survivors surveying the wreckage of downed trees, ruined buildings, and dashed hopes.

If your anger escalates rapidly like a tropical storm gathering over a warm ocean, or if you're like a tinderbox, ready to ignite at the slightest provocation, you're probably aware of the damage it's causing. Your spouse is cautious around you and scared of setting you off by not talking anymore. Your children instinctively avoid you, running helter-skelter like white mice, scared that the slightest infraction—an unwashed plate, dirty shoes, messy homework, or a neglected chore—will turn you into a raging inferno. Sometimes, no one will say anything, but they'll start finding excuses not to be around you—and avoid you when your paths cross. When it's your spouse or your children doing this, you might need to take stock before the most critical relationships in your life shatter on the rocky shores of your rage.

A father facing this predicament commented on a YouTube video, "I know my relationship with my two daughters is at risk because of my anger issues. My outbursts are also escalating, becoming more violent, and it's really bothering me."

Another said, "I've been having problems with anger for a while. I often lash out at my family, sometimes over trivial things. I get angry when people disagree with me too."

You might know intuitively that something is wrong but cannot extricate yourself. As one mother told me, "Everything is a trigger. I've come to realize that my overwhelming need to control everything has ruined my relationships with my family and friends. Everyone I know seems to be afraid of me."

Perhaps your children, unconsciously mimicking you, have developed their own angry responses to people and situations. On social media, an exhausted mother says with vague bewilderment, "My children always fight. They're incredibly jealous and competitive, and they're constantly angry with each other. Unfortunately, this triggers me too."

Another woman adds, "My daughter insists on correcting everything I do and say. I'm a naturally angry person, and I can see that she's the same. I am very concerned. I don't want her to grow up like this."

THE MYTH OF THE "GOOD PARENT"

There's a palpable excitement from the moment your pregnancy is confirmed. Will you have a boy or a girl—or do you want to be surprised? Which room in your home will be the nursery? As your bump grows, you'll be investing in this tiny new life—decorating the nursery, and buying baby clothes, furniture, diapers, pacifiers, bibs, and soft toys. You'll read books on babies and childcare, burning up the internet to find out everything you can before the happy event. You'll identify with women pushing strollers or leading toddlers by the hand through parks or across busy city streets. You'll think about how you'll raise your beautiful human and what kind of a person they'll become.

Of course, you'll want to be the perfect parent, like the ones pictured in the baby and parenting magazines—happy, smiling, and calm no matter what life (or your child) throws at you, building a wonderful relationship with this little person. You might naturally be a perfectionist, or you will immerse yourself and the subtle societal pressure to become the ideal mom—or dad. The media is full of pictures, videos, and movies showing cooing babies and cute, smiling toddlers with serenely attractive mothers and fathers.

But the truth is that we're not perfect, and neither is the world we live in. Have you ever found yourself parenting reactively, snapping at your kids, and barely keeping the peace? At these times, especially if this happens often, you might wonder if you're a terrible parent. Parenting is a challenging job that society seems to notice or reward barely. Most of us have no idea of what's involved until we have our own children. Let's face it: Parenting is hard, challenging work.

Having said that, it's not necessary to compare yourself with other parents and imagine that their journey is less chaotic than yours. Young children especially let it all hang out. They don't notice whether their parents are more put together than those of the little guy they sit next to in kindergarten. They don't fuss about designer clothes, perfect houses, or the ideal family car. They are who they are, and they make their feelings about the world known. All parents are in the same boat, so to speak, no matter how things might appear to outsiders.

Caring for and guiding another human being is an essential journey that many of us make—one for which we're given little or no training. There are late nights, early mornings, and midnight feeds, mysterious ailments, teething, finicky eaters, and a newly walking child suddenly having access to things that were once beyond their reach. It can be a little daunting, having someone totally dependent on you for everything. But it can also be beautiful, with those innocent, wonderful moments when you're so happy to be a mother or father.

You'll be tired, too, especially if you're working full-time, and you'll still have the usual stresses and responsibilities of everyday life to deal with in addition to child-rearing. And sometimes there'll be tantrums, backchat, cheekiness, and stubbornness to deal with, depending on your child's character—or your child may simply seem to have their own agenda, which might not coincide with yours.

It can be hard to keep your cool when your child is uncooperative, and you're under stress, even if it's something simple like the possibility of you being late for work or having your daily commute derailed first thing in the morning. And especially if you come from a family of angry people—or even if you don't—your first reaction to the discomfort and helplessness you feel might be to get angry, to start yelling and shouting, or to punish your kids out of all proportion to the actual situation.

Bear in mind that anger can be contagious: if one parent becomes angry regularly, chances are that the spouse will also pick up this behavior. This means that there will ultimately be no peace in the home.

One woman explained this on social media based on her own experience. "I did not battle with anger until my children were born—although my husband often struggled to control his temper. Eventually, I found myself being triggered as well. The trouble is that we're both proud and stubborn. We have huge fights where neither of us wants to give in. We each believe we're right—but we're actually both wrong."

CONTROLLING YOUR ANGER BEFORE IT CONTROLS YOU

If you find that you're developing anger issues—and especially if it's getting more intense and starting to control you—you need to deal with the problem without delay. Don't get me wrong: There's nothing wrong with emotions, including anger. Emotions are part of being human. They enable us to express ourselves, respond to our world and one another, and enjoy a fulfilled life enhanced by positive, enriching relationships with others. Anger becomes a problem when it gets out of hand, when it's an instantaneous, knee-jerk response to any adverse situation, no matter how trivial, and when we're constantly taking out our frustrations on everyone around us. (Perhaps some of you reading this book are already seeing this in your own lives.)

While experiencing angry emotions isn't wrong, the crux of the matter is how you deal with them—or don't. This is such a powerful emotion that we need to ensure that it doesn't rule us. Even Saint Paul, writing to the church in Ephesus, advised his readers, "Do not let your anger lead you into sin: Do not let the sun go down while you are still angry." (Ephesians 4:26) (Holy Bible, New International Version, 1974).

Believe it or not, succumbing to anger is a choice, and it needs to be dealt with just like any other "negative" emotion. We need to harness our feelings rather than let them hold us captive in a destructive cycle. Dealing with our feelings constructively and expressing anger in a controlled, logical way doesn't come naturally—it's a skill that needs to be learned.

Anger can be a reflection of ourselves. It's indicative of how we perceive the world and respond to it. People get angry for a host of reasons. Anger can be sparked by things such as fear, insecurity, frustration, or feelings of inadequacy or helplessness, for example. The reasons why we fly off the handle with little apparent cause can be very deep-seated. You're also more likely to be an angry person if your parents were angry people. If you've grown up in a mad household, where everyone was yelling and shouting, you may not even know what it is to build an oasis of calm in your home.

But none of this is any excuse. Our children are not responsible for our past hurts, current circumstances, or feelings. We shouldn't take out our emotions on them inappropriately. Did you know that if you're a parent who is inclined to yell at your children, you could actually be training them to ignore you? Yelling might not only subtly encourage your children's bad behavior, but it could also damage their mental health and young brains.

If you're in that situation and you're reading this book, that's a good thing. It means you've recognized the problem, and you're taking charge of it, so you don't raise angry people. You've started on the path to healing and wholeness by becoming aware that something is wrong.

In this book, I will discuss the various faces of anger and how to cope with this fierce emotion. I'll explain how you can determine where the fury stems from, how to recognize your triggers, and how to deal with them, so the anger you feel doesn't destroy your life. I'll show you how to come to terms with anger as a parent and how to avoid raising people who are as mad at the world as you are. (Hopefully, you'll be a little less furious after reading this book.)

1

UNDERSTANDING YOUR ANGER

> *Holding onto anger is like grasping a hot coal with the intention of throwing it at someone else; you are the one who gets burned.*
>
> — BUDDHA

Everyone gets angry. A traffic snarl-up threatens to make you late for an appointment. You finally get onto the highway to find yourself stuck behind someone driving too slowly—and you can't pass because there's too much traffic traveling at regular highway speeds in the other lanes. You start fuming, thinking to yourself that people who drive like this shouldn't be allowed on freeways or even given a license.

Your boss picks you out in front of your colleagues. You're outraged, but you don't say anything then. After all, he's your superior. Over lunch, you complain to a friend, "He was so disrespectful! How could he speak to me like that in front of everyone?"

It's essential to recognize at the outset that anger is a normal, healthy emotion. It's not a mental illness. Most people, in fact, get angry at times, but their emotions are manageable, and it hardly causes a ripple in their lives. So, precisely what is this fierce, potentially explosive emotion that makes your heart race and your blood boil?

The American Psychological Association defines anger as "an emotion characterized by antagonism toward someone, or something you feel has deliberately done you wrong" (American Psychological Association, n.d.). The association says that about 25% of anger incidents involve vengeful thoughts to "get even" or "put them in their place" (American Psychological Association, 2021).

To be clear, anger isn't the same as aggression, although the two might be linked. Anger is a negative emotion characterized by hostility, psychological arousal, and antisocial behaviors. Angry thoughts can tense your muscles, give you headaches, or increase your heart rate. Anger is often expressed verbally through shouting, arguing, swearing—and even being sarcastic. It might be accompanied by physical actions, such as throwing or hitting objects, or raising a clenched fist.

Aggression, on the other hand, is underpinned by a desire for control and domination, and aggressive people often hurt others intentionally. Such behavior can include physical threats, sometimes with a weapon. Aggression is typically associated with domestic violence, child or elder abuse, bullying, or criminal activities.

Loud verbal outbursts are typical of anger, but only 10% of these culminate in aggression. By contrast, 90% of aggressive incidents are preceded by anger (American Psychological Association, 2021). Anger on its own is unlikely to get you in trouble with the law, but anger that results in aggression—or is fueled by it—probably will.

Often referred to as a secondary emotion, anger is complex, frequently spurred by other feelings, with fear, sadness, or disgust lurking beneath the fury, like some psychological Loch Ness monster. We nearly always feel something else before we get angry. If these feelings are intense enough, we perceive the entire emotion as anger. A good example is when someone cuts us off while driving in heavy traffic. Most of us immediately feel angry. Almost no one recognizes that in that millisecond before we sounded the horn or took evasive action, we felt a spurt of fear that our physical safety could be jeopardized by a vehicle accident. In reality, anger is like an iceberg (see diagram below) in that only some emotions are apparent. The vast majority are hidden below the waterline, where they are not immediately obvious to others—or even to us.

Anger

disgusted anxious annoyed frustrated
rejected scared jealous attacked
guilt embarrassed Sad insecure
hungry worried disappointed hurt
trapped tired ashamed helpless

Angry outbursts very often have fear, vulnerability, or personal insecurity at their core. These can all be overcome by self-confidence. If you have good self-esteem, you need not fear changing circumstances. You won't worry about what others think if you have a clear conscience. If you trust in your skills or efforts and know you are doing your best, you don't need to be jealous. If you know you have value as a person—whether you believe that you are a child of God or are just a good human being—then you will be more likely to ignore other people's offensiveness.

I personally realized that I am at my best when I'm not responding to situations out of fear. Once the fear is addressed, the anger is considerably diminished. It might even disappear entirely.

However, it's also important not to bottle up your emotions. Otherwise, the anger builds up and will explode one day. If your anger is out of control and hurting those around you, then it's a problem.

UNCONTROLLED ANGER

If not adequately managed, anger can negatively affect you and those around you. When you're angry, you might find yourself doing or saying things that you regret once the outburst is over. You can make serious mistakes when you are blindly mad. Anger can hurt you mentally and physically and potentially damage your most important relationships. It's not a good idea to use alcohol or drugs to deal with anger—it may make things even worse.

There are several ways to identify whether your anger is getting out of control. These include:

- Your anger usually manifests in unhelpful or destructive behavior.
- It is negatively affecting your mental and physical health.
- Anger dominates you, frequently blotting out all other feelings and emotions.
- You can't seem to express your anger in healthy, constructive ways.

There are, sadly, many unhealthy, unhelpful, and often isolating ways of expressing anger. You may become outwardly aggressive and violent. You might shout, swear, slam doors, hit or throw things, and become physically violent, verbally abusive, or threatening towards others. This behavior can be extremely frightening and psychologically damaging for those around you, especially children. This is a hazardous way to express your anger. You may end up losing your family —or find yourself in trouble with the law. If you find that your anger is escalating to this point, it's critical to seek help and support as soon as possible.

But not all extreme anger manifests in such a physical, frightening way. A more subtle form of expressing anger includes ignoring people and stonewalling them. You may refuse to do certain chores and tasks, or do them badly or at the last minute, frustrating others. You might sulk, never expressing your anger explicitly or aggressively.

Anger can also be turned inwards. You could convince yourself that you are a hateful person. You might deny yourself basic needs, such as food or things that might make you happy. You may cut yourself off from the world or even do self-harm.

If you find that you are struggling with anger, you must address the issue promptly. Anger is a powerful, potentially dangerous emotion. The more you give in to it and allow it to manifest, the more intense it will become. It makes no difference whether your anger is the explosive kind, the quiet "freeze you out" sort, or is turning inwards to erode your personality from the inside; the result is the same.

Anger builds up over time if your feelings aren't mitigated when something happens that triggers you. A series of minor daily irritations can lead to a meltdown over something simple. If you've had a long, frustrating day when everything seems to be against you, a minor incident—mislaying a credit card, tripping over a toy, or a broken shopping bag—can trigger an explosion. This happens because all the minor irritations of the day weren't dealt with appropriately when they happened, hence the furious outburst.

WHERE DOES ANGER COME FROM?

Anger is one of the five basic emotions—anger, fear, sadness, disgust, and enjoyment—that are found in most human cultures (Center for Clinical Psychology, n.d.). These emotions appear in early childhood and are believed to be a substitute for the survival instincts found in most living creatures. Emotions such as anger and fear alert us to dangerous situations that could harm us.

Our senses constantly monitor the surrounding environment for potential threats. When one is detected, a message is sent to the amygdala in the brain, which is associated with emotions like fear, anxiety, and anger. This prepares the body for a fight-or-flight response. This is entirely unconscious and is how anger is created biologically.

After this, another message is transmitted to the cerebral cortex—the part of the brain that processes our thoughts. We evaluate the nature of the threat and decide what we want to do about it if anything. This is the reaction part of anger. The fight-or-flight response is triggered if we decide that an aggressive or hostile reaction is required.

The fight-or-flight response is when our bodies react to threatening situations by releasing hormones like adrenaline and cortisol. Cortisol is manufactured and released by the adrenal cortex, the outermost section of the adrenal glands, which are located above the kidneys. Hormones like adrenaline (or epinephrine) are substances known as catecholamines produced by the adrenal medulla in the brain and some nerve fibers. Adrenaline rapidly increases the heart rate, respiration, and other subtle changes in the body.

Cortisol is released more slowly over hours or days. The hormone norepinephrine signals its release to prepare the body for long-term stress. Cortisol inhibits growth and reproduction and changes the body's metabolism to enable either quick action or future famine by raising blood sugar levels and increasing fat storage.

These biological reactions alert us and speed up our reaction time, and they limit blood flow to the torso and send it to the arms and legs, where it would be most needed to run away from an enemy or other threat. Breathing, heart rate, blood pressure, and body temperature also increase. This is when our anger erupts, sometimes volcanically.

Our brain chemistry reflects our emotions. Cortisol decreases when we are consumed by happy thoughts or feel joy, and the brain releases serotonin in response to our positive emotions. When serotonin levels are optimal, we feel calmer, more comfortable, more focused, and more emotionally stable.

UNCONTROLLED ANGER MAY DAMAGE YOUR HEALTH

Uncontrolled anger, hostility, and rage are a ticking time bomb for your body. Medical research has shown that excessive anger can negatively impact your health, sometimes exacerbating existing health issues.

Specific health problems might also contribute to anger, creating a vicious circle. People suffering from dementia and conditions like Alzheimer's sometimes experience heightened levels of anger and aggression. Some anti-anxiety drugs, sleeping pills, and cholesterol-lowering medication can increase anger responses in patients. The cholesterol-lowering medication also reduces serotonin levels, increasing irritability. People with diabetes, especially those suffering from low blood sugar, are more likely to become angry because the same hormones regulate glucose levels and stress. Women undergoing premenstrual syndrome (PMS) or menopause sometimes become angrier as hormonal changes disturb serotonin levels. An overactive thyroid may also increase tension and irritability but can be improved with medication.

This creates a problem: you can't sort out your mental state until you resolve the health problem, but you also can't do that until you cool off, give yourself space, and stay away from the things that trigger your anger. There's nothing wrong with being a hermit for a while in the interests of your overall mental and physical well-being.

Common Health Problems Associated with Uncontrolled Anger

Liver Problems

People with chronic liver disease are often very irritable and angry. Traditional Chinese Medicine (TCM) practitioners have long believed that anger blocks the liver's energy flow, damaging this vital organ. This view has subsequently been confirmed by medical research. When the liver fails, it cannot remove toxins from the body. This ultimately causes a brain disorder, resulting in personality changes and an inability to regulate one's emotions.

Duke University Medical Center researchers found that otherwise healthy people prone to anger produce higher levels of the C-reactive protein (CRP) usually produced by the liver in response to inflammation (Cutler, 2011). CRP is implicated in cardiovascular disease and strokes. Additional research on patients undergoing treatment for hepatitis C, which may cause chronic liver damage, found that patients were angrier during treatment than average (Cutler, 2011). This also harmed the liver, creating a vicious circle. Several other studies have established that stress-related emotions could damage the liver.

Cardiovascular Disease and Strokes

As previously mentioned, when you are angry, your body initiates the fight-or-flight response, producing hormones such as cortisol and catecholamines. Among other things, these raise your heart rate and breathing, giving you energy. They also tighten your blood vessels, so your blood pressure increases. If this happens often, this causes wear and tear on your artery walls.

Studies investigating the links between certain personality traits and the development of coronary artery disease (CAD) established that hostility signals, including anger, cynicism, and mistrust, may contribute to the development of CAD, as well as an increased likelihood of fatal heart attacks (Rozanski et al., 1999). Hostility is often associated with unhealthy lifestyles characterized by smoking, poor diet, obesity, and alcoholism. Contentious subjects generally had higher heart rates and blood pressure when performing mental tasks and higher blood pressure in general. Low levels of perceived emotional support also increase the risk of CAD.

Stomach Upsets and Lack of Appetite

The body's fight-or-flight mechanism reduces blood flow to the gut. When you experience long-term stress, the production of cortisol undermines the immune system and suppresses digestion and the reproductive system, as well as stunting growth processes.

Eczema and Skin Problems

Did you know that your skin is more prone to wrinkles if you are always angry? That's because the high levels of cortisol present in angry people inhibit the production of collagen, a crucial element in skin healing. When collagen production slows, wrinkles result. One study found that healing and cell turnover took as much as four times longer in angry participants compared to those with calmer dispositions (Gold, 2013).

Lung Problems

There is evidence that negative emotions might be associated with chronic airway obstruction. A study published in 2006 established a definite correlation between hostility and reduced lung function, even after allowing for factors such as smoking and education (Kubzansky et al., 2006). Higher hostility sped up the decline.

Other Problems

Hostile, angry responses to the world, in general, are also associated with headaches, memory loss, insomnia, depression, and fatigue. Anger is particularly harmful to pregnant or breastfeeding women.

PSYCHOLOGICAL EFFECTS OF ANGER

Anger, especially unresolved, may precipitate faulty thinking patterns, such as believing in "all or nothing" or "either-or," without allowing for any middle ground or gradient. This means that people might end up divided into two camps, as is happening increasingly in the United States and worldwide due to the COVID pandemic. Finding the middle ground prevents polarization and increases mental flexibility.

Unresolved anger creates attribution biases, in other words, incorrect assumptions about the beliefs or actions of other people. For example, one might not understand someone else's situation but will nevertheless draw conclusions about their character that might be flawed or even wholly unfounded. Anger has also been found to reduce tolerance.

POSITIVE ASPECTS OF ANGER

Surprisingly, anger isn't necessarily destructive. Feeling angry is usually a good indicator that something is wrong. It can be a positive emotion in that it helps us see things clearly, enabling us to identify hurting or harmful situations. Anger positively expressed can motivate us to change our circumstances, achieve our goals, and transform our lives.

Anger ensures that others listen to us and that our voices are heard. It alerts others to the fact that we feel agitated and uncomfortable. It may force others to improve their actions towards us. Asserting that you were first in line at a store could encourage better service, for instance. Anger can help ensure better outcomes in business negotiations if one of the parties feels strongly about a particular issue. Anger as a response to injustice tends to spur social change. An excellent example of this is slavery. The practice would never have been abolished if people like Abraham Lincoln and William Wilberforce hadn't become angry about how other human beings were being treated.

PARENTAL ANGER

Hurricane mom or dad must realize that we don't live like wolves in the tundra. The triggers we get from our children aren't real threats, so we shouldn't react. Parental anger does not have to be expressed by a volcanic eruption but can be a simple statement of fact. You could tell your children something has made you angry or disappointed without yelling. Shouting and acting out your anger is probably one of the worst ways to express this powerful emotion with your children—and it can even damage their brains.

Research conducted at McLean Hospital found that verbal abuse from parents and friends causes detrimental changes in developing brains—and the effects can last into adulthood (Dougherty, 2022). Exposure to verbal abuse can be similar to witnessing domestic and other forms of violence or even experiencing sexual assault. The study found that specific neural pathways in adults subjected to verbal abuse as children were disturbed. Verbal abuse may lead to negative emotions finding expression in physical illness. It might even raise the likelihood of drug abuse, anxiety, and depression in teens, as well as increased anger and hostility in young adults.

2

WHAT MAKES YOU AN ANGRY PARENT? ALL ABOUT TRIGGERS

> *Every day we have plenty of opportunities to get angry, stressed, or offended. But what you're doing when you indulge these negative emotions is giving something outside of yourself power over your happiness. You can choose not to let little things upset you.*
>
> — JOEL OSTEEN

One of the most pervasive triggers for anger in the U.S. today is directly attributable to the COVID pandemic. While everyone was locked away—and in the subsequent return to our new normal—it seemed that our collective anger was festering. We were frustrated. Our daily routines were disrupted entirely. We could no longer go to work and interact with our colleagues in a normal fashion, having meetings, lunches, conferences—or even chats at the coffee machine. We had to settle for online meetings instead, sometimes still in our pajamas and while being interrupted by our children, spouses, or pets. Despite the humorous videos and advertisements that emerged from the experience, not being able to interact normally was incredibly frustrating. After that, so many people decided not to return to their former employment that the phenomenon known as the Great Resignation arose, with people resigning from their jobs in droves.

Lockdowns and the hesitant return to "normal" weren't particularly easy on children and teens either. A family member with a teenage daughter told me, "They can chat online on their phones, of course, but it's just not the same. They miss being with their friends, hanging out on the beach, and doing things together." As schools across the world closed, many parents, who were already trying to balance online work and offline chores and activities to avoid the whole family coming down with a severe case of cabin fever, suddenly found themselves homeschooling. While there's nothing wrong with homeschooling, being forced into it was more than many parents had bargained on. It was yet another responsibility that had to be done.

The frustration, resentment, and powerlessness we all collectively felt, especially as the pandemic dragged on, had nowhere to go. This meant that the pandemic effectively incubated the anger many were feeling—and still are, as we struggle with our altered circumstances and those of the societies in which we live. It's gotten so bad that it's even got a name: Pandemic rage.

A *New York Times* article cites some telling examples. There was the exhausted restaurant owner battling supply and staff shortages who had customers angry at the slow service of ordering an entire meal, only to dump the whole thing, very publicly, in the garbage. Then there was the airline passenger who got so drunk and abusive that the terrified flight attendants eventually duct-taped him to his seat. (That sounds funny at first glance, but flight attendants increasingly report that passengers look right through them as though they don't exist.) Shop attendants across the country are increasingly subjected to verbal abuse when items are unavailable. Everyone is frustrated and on edge.

An article by Travis D. Westbrook from Ohio State University's Wexner Medical Center suggests that we've all developed such hair-trigger tempers since the advent of the pandemic stress, which increases frustration and irritability. The article, written in 2020, says that our everyday lives suddenly and quickly became more complicated, and activities that might have helped us deal with the stress were curtailed (Westbrook, 2020). So, instead of enjoying a social evening or running, people started lashing out at friends, especially family, to relieve stress and frustration.

According to the Mayo Clinic, mental fatigue has now set in. People are experiencing depression, anxiety, and anger that never entirely go away. Pandemic anger—or "panger"—is something people are increasingly grappling with.

Parents are especially vulnerable to something triggering their anger, as children are naturally inclined to find the chinks in their psyche—and have been doing since they were in diapers.

MANAGING EXPECTATIONS

For starters, you need to take it as a given that your children will push your buttons. They will only sometimes do what you want them to do when you want them to do it. This can spark your anger if you are so inclined. Children are, in fact, supposed to push against the boundaries set for them to find out who they are and ultimately establish their own identities. However, knowing this doesn't make it any easier when you feel you are being tested or ignored, as the case may be. The best policy is not only to expect it but also to accept it. This will help you keep calm. It's still important to establish boundaries and ensure that your children know what these are—and that it's their responsibility to adhere to them.

Some parents need clarification as to what they are responsible for and what their children are responsible for. Remember that your child will have responsibilities in life that they need to adhere to. If you feel that you need to control how things turn out, you will stunt your child's growth and frustrate them, which ultimately spawns more stress and anxiety for everyone. In addition, if you're always solving your children's problems, as opposed to teaching them how to solve their own, they will expect you to do that all the time. This will eventually overburden you, making you stressed, anxious, and frustrated. It's not good for your child either.

Parents need to teach their children good life and relationship skills, establish rules for family life, and ensure effective consequences if their children don't adhere to behavioral boundaries. But the rest is up to your child.

Don't fall into the trap of living in the future, worrying about whether your children will always be like they are now and whether they can manage as adults. This type of thinking can undermine your ability to parent effectively. Psychologists refer to this as "thinking errors," where your thoughts don't align with reality and are inclined to be negative and self-defeating. Please don't assume the worst: It very likely won't happen anyway.

Be prepared, so you aren't ambushed by your own anxiety or how others could respond to you. Sometimes you know from experience that there's going to be a conflict because, for example, your teenager nearly always comes home from school in a rebellious mood, or you're going to need to say "no" to one of your children's requests, which they won't like. Decide in advance that you're not going to get into an argument. Once again, don't allow your children to press your buttons.

ANGER'S TRIGGERS

A trigger, loosely speaking, is something that evokes an emotional response in you when someone does something that makes you react. This reaction can sometimes be positive, but it can also be negative, like when it provokes an angry outburst on your side, mainly when dealing with your child.

Some indications that you've been triggered include the following:

- any time you find yourself excessively angry with your children,
- if you're unusually sad or hurt after your child or spouse says or does something you know you shouldn't take personally,
- if your feelings are out of proportion to the situation or out of control,
- if the feelings seem to be explosive and come out of nowhere,
- if you find yourself suddenly wanting to hurt your child physically.

Being able to identify your triggers and understanding the emotions behind them is crucial in helping you manage your anger. While most authorities lump together all anger triggers, I feel it's more helpful to separate them into what I'll call "visible triggers" and "invisible triggers."

Visible Triggers

Visible triggers are situations or events that make us feel threatened, attacked, frustrated, disrespected, powerless, or that we're being mistreated. You will likely become angry if someone belittles you or does not respect you or your possessions.

Other triggers we need to deal with these days are those related to the inconvenience and heightened scrutiny we're all experiencing due to COVID. You might constantly be moving from working at the office to working from home when someone at work tests positive for the virus. Your boss has started expecting everyone to be available at all hours for online meetings, disrupting your family time. Friends might have criticized your decision not to wear a mask in public, although the authorities have allowed this. A much-anticipated holiday may have had to be canceled because someone in your party unexpectedly tested positive for COVID. Your child's grades might not have recovered after a prolonged stint of online learning, and they feel pressured and resentful.

Common parenting triggers include crying, whining, tantrums, disobedience, non-compliance, passive resistance, sibling fighting, or anything your child does that makes you angry or upset. You might be triggered if your two-year-old is a constant whiner at home, your daughter gets upset at her younger brother (who is actually annoying everyone), or your son throws a temper tantrum at a friend's birthday party.

People interpret things differently, so something that makes one person incredibly angry may not provoke another. If you're a parent, you're bound to have experienced a situation where your child did something that made you mad while your spouse saw the humor in the case. It's important to remember that it doesn't mean that you have misinterpreted a situation if you become angry, but someone else doesn't.

How you react to a particular situation or set of circumstances depends on several factors, including your life experiences. These are what I prefer to call "invisible triggers."

Invisible Triggers

Dan Siegel, in his book *Parenting From the Inside Out*, has this in mind when he writes, "Issues that are rooted in our past impact our present reality and directly affect the way we experience and interact with our children, even when we're unaware of their origins" (Siegel, 2005).

Because anger is such a complex emotion, often caused by other emotions—and frequently exacerbated by stress, frustration, or everyday life experiences—there may be several reasons you're having difficulty expressing your anger positively and constructively.

Visible triggers often invoke the invisible ones, and that could be why you might find yourself becoming excessively angry over trivial things. If you don't address these invisible triggers, a minor incident is enough to send you into overdrive. Take the situation with my daughter. I have a tough time trying not to get angry with her. Due to COVID, I'm routinely working from home, but my daughter and her cousins make a lot of noise when they get together at our place, which is most days. What really gets me going is when they continue whispering and giggling even after I have asked them to keep quiet because I have an online meeting.

In another scenario, your child flatly refuses to cooperate. That takes you back to your own childhood, and you again feel some measure of the helplessness you experienced when you were not allowed to express your emotions. All that old hurt and anger comes bubbling up from your subconscious—because it hasn't been resolved. However, this time, it gets directed at your child instead of the person who upset you in the past.

Many triggers come from our childhood experiences in our own families and with our parents as we were growing up. If you had parents who were constantly yelling at you and abusive towards you, you might suffer from insecurity because of low self-esteem. This could drive you to lash out in anger or rage. You may not even be aware on a conscious level that this is happening.

For instance, your daughter, who is in third grade, comes to you for help with some math homework. It's been a long day for you, and you are tired. When you look at it, you see that she made the same mistake with a problem you painstakingly taught her just a few days ago. So, you blow up and say something you regret later. However, your fierce reaction frightened your daughter, who cried a lot after the incident. The takeaway from this scenario is not to try and tutor your children when you are tired or hungry. Based on experience, you know their dependence on you is more likely to make you mad when you are exhausted.

Your Childhood and Upbringing

A psychotherapist friend—who has been conducting therapy for over 25 years—says that, in her experience, most of her client's problems originate in much earlier unresolved life events and traumas. The mind and body cry out as we spiral into depression, anxiety, neuroses, and physical illness.

As children, we can easily be hurt and controlled by our parents and siblings, together with other adults we might interact with. At the time, we couldn't defend ourselves, and we might have been prevented from openly expressing our feelings. In extreme cases, we could not physically flee from verbal or physical abuse or neglect. We, therefore, develop coping mechanisms or defenses to help us survive our families. While these were appropriate at the time, we might still use them as adults. In addition, our experiences have likely left behind several emotional loose ends.

Suppose you were excessively punished when you disobeyed your parents. In that case, you may be triggered when your child challenges you—or when your child says something decisive that takes you back to when you were a frightened, insecure, resentful, or helpless child.

You might not have been allowed to express your emotions when you were a child without being ridiculed in some way, and you may become angry when your child is upset because you see echoes of your younger self. Many men, growing up, were not allowed to cry, so they found it very hard to hear a crying child. They may become angry to cover up their unease.

As a child, you may have observed anger playing out so that it's harder for you to deal with your fury as an adult. If you often get angry quickly and explosively, you may have grown up in a family where anger was expressed aggressively or violently. Hence, you have yet to learn how to understand or manage your feelings.

You may have had first-hand exposure to the consequences of out-of-control adult anger and come to believe that all anger is destructive and terrifying. You might be afraid of it and don't feel safe expressing your feelings when you're annoyed or upset. However, these emotions can't stay bottled up and may surface after the event has passed, bewildering you and others.

You might have been punished for being angry or brought up to believe that you shouldn't complain. As an adult, you might be suppressing your anger. This may mean that you inappropriately react when you feel uncomfortable or are exposed to new situations. Without a healthy way to express it, anger could turn inwards.

Traumatic Past Experiences

You might be coping with historic anger caused by past events. These could include being abused or bullied as a child or adult or having undergone some other traumatic experience. This could mean that certain situations have the potential to make you unreasonably angry. Sometimes, the anger you feel at these times is compounded by the unresolved anger from your past. This leads you to respond way out of proportion to the current situation. Resolving your history can enable you to react to present triggers in a safer, more appropriate way.

Current Circumstances

If you're dealing with many other problems in life, your anger might be triggered more frequently. You're more likely to become angry when you're tired, hungry, overwhelmed, or stressed. One of the signs of this kind of stress is when trivial, unrelated things make you angry. This often happens if you cannot resolve your anger around a given situation.

COMMON CHALLENGES FOR SHORT-FUSED PARENTS

You may feel that, as a parent, you have a temper that arrives suddenly, like a lightning flash. Before you know it, you're like an enraged bull at a bullfight, charging into the ring and ready to do severe damage. But your rage is frequently out of proportion to the actual event that triggered it. Perhaps your child lost her swimming costume on a school outing, did poorly in a math test, or got home later than expected after seeing friends on the weekend.

People who feel insecure are more likely to get volcanically angry at short notice. Fury is a defense mechanism against low self-esteem for those who haven't developed the ability to express their feelings more positively. Their fears—that their inadequacy will be revealed or that they will be ridiculed—makes them lash out with angry outbursts and explosive rage, often alarming or frightening those around them.

Irritability is frequently a sign of stress, unhappiness, or both. When people are under significant pressure—or believe they are—it's often "that one little thing" that pushes them over the edge, and they lash out. It's worth remembering, especially if you're the one on the receiving end, that angrily lashing out is the easy way out instead of taking a deep breath, addressing one's feelings, and getting to the root of the problem. To think of it, inherently happy people don't get angry very easily, while relaxed individuals rarely get upset over trivialities.

Another reason why people exhibit explosive behavior is when they're unable to compromise. There can be many reasons for this, but usually, they were never taught to do so. They might have had overly indulgent parents—or hard, inflexible ones, who denied their child's every request. An unremitting "yes" or "no" to every appeal a child makes ultimately teaches them to view the world in terms of black or white, where they either get everything or nothing from it.

Intolerance is another characteristic of those who get angry quickly and violently. Most situations can be worked out. However, some outraged people never realize this until late in life—and sometimes never. Based on my observations, people who tend to overthink everything or have very calculating personalities are easily angered.

Uncontrolled anger is a sign of poor self-control, and those who regularly vent their fury on others give in to their angry feelings. Often it's not merely anger that they feel but the much more destructive, distilled version of it—rage. For example, people prone to road rage aren't angry so much as being completely out of control.

CONTROLLING YOUR TEMPER AS A PARENT

Children have minds of their own. They don't always behave the way you would like them to. Toddlers are apt to have tantrums in the check-out queue at the supermarket at the end of the month when the place is the busiest. Your teenage daughter is finding her place in the world and gets annoyed when you tell her that she must be back from a weekend outing by a specific time: She tells you that none of her friends have a curfew for that evening. These scenarios—and hundreds like them in the daily task of child-raising—can provoke an angry response in you. The key is recognizing what's happening and disconnecting your emotional reaction from your child's actions. If you react emotionally, you create boundaries about what is safe and not safe for your kids to talk to you about.

There is no qualification for parenthood and no approved or accredited way to become a good parent. There are no colleges or universities offering parenthood diplomas or degrees. We're all winging it by trial and error.

Researching the different developmental stages of a child—and what to expect in each phase—can help educate and prepare you so that you are not taken by surprise when your child acts in a certain way. Even though you'll need to iron out a lot of the details as you go along, this will help you to understand what is happening to your child, so you can be supportive and guide them wisely, as opposed to simply reacting, often inappropriately. (To assist you, I'll cover some aspects of this topic in the next chapter.)

Certain life stages, like the so-called "terrible twos" or the emotional roller-coaster exhibited by teenagers, can be explained by physical changes, such as the brain developing or hormones becoming active. Tantrums of one kind or another may be part of these life stages, although the temper two-year-old throws will be quite different from that of a teenager shouting at you and slamming their bedroom door in your face.

Children usually throw continuous tantrums because they have been trained to do so. Their parents might have spoiled them, so they throw a tantrum if they cannot have what they desire or do what they like. The child has learned from experience that doing this elicits the action or reaction they want and that they can manipulate others.

It can be tough to remain calm when your toddler begins whining and crying, keeping this up for a long time. Eventually, your temper flares, and your patience goes out the window. If your child's crying regularly triggers your anger, consider whether something in your past could make this happen. For example, you might have been told to "shut up" whenever you cried as a child. Once you understand why it bothers you,

you will find it easier to control your emotional reaction to these behaviors.

Sibling rivalry can be another trigger. You might become angry, too, and start to side with one or the other of your warring children. Again, it's essential to step back from the situation and ask yourself why their argument or fight is upsetting you so much that you can't distance yourself from it.

Other things your children do may upset you to the point where you start responding inappropriately. Consider all these when evaluating your reactions.

MANAGING YOUR TRIGGERS

Begin by making it a habit to write down all the things that elicited angry responses from you during the day and what triggered them. Remember to make a note of how you handled a particular trigger. Update the list regularly to monitor your progress and see whether you're improving.

Anger management is an emotional skill you need to practice even when you're not angry, which brings us to the concept of "self-mindfulness." Ask yourself questions like these: "Does getting angry make me feel happy?" "Will getting angry improve my health?" If the answer to such questions is a resounding "no," why do you continue doing it?

If you make an effort to cultivate such mindfulness, it will eventually become part of your everyday repertoire of psychological skills. When you are conscious and aware during an anger-generating incident, you will be able to understand what is happening, regulate your reactions, and ultimately subdue your anger.

3

LOVE YOURSELF—AND MITIGATE INVISIBLE TRIGGERS

> *If you choose yourself above all and develop an immense love for yourself, nothing could make you sad.*
>
> — ANON

It's natural to put our children first once we become parents. That's what good parents do, after all. However, we often overlook one simple fact: Only when we can take diligent care of ourselves can we take good care of children. We are their cornerstones. Our children are not able to look after us, so we need to be the ones who take good care of ourselves. This makes us better parents too.

We need to acknowledge that we can't always control our children's behavior—but we can control our reactions to it. We can't change other people, but we can change ourselves. If we care for ourselves and love ourselves, we're much less likely to lose our tempers as parents.

SEEKING HELP

Surprisingly, depression and even sadness can often lurk beneath intensely angry outbursts. This is particularly true for men, who find it challenging to express emotions like sadness. We need to acknowledge the full range of our feelings and talk them through with another person—a therapist or trusted friend. This is a big part of anger management.

Anger can also indicate old hurts that occurred long ago and still need to be worked through. Consider taking part in wellness therapy, which has both a physical and emotional aspect, to address these niggling hurts. A therapist will analyze your shortcomings and give you a structured approach to work through each one. Alternatively, you can join a community comprised of those who have had similar experiences. This will not only make you feel complete, but it will also help you love yourself. If you don't seek help addressing underlying issues, it might be tough to manage your anger due to an invisible trigger.

Be kind to yourself. There are several things you can do to increase your happiness. Here are a few surprisingly simple ones:

- Take ten deep breaths. This may sound quaint, but it will force you to slow down and relax. It takes only two minutes but sends a strong message to the brain to calm down (King, 2020). It also loosens all tense muscles and untangles your thoughts. It's a great way to relieve stress during a hectic day.
- Remember to smile. There's a good biological reason why smiling is both good for you and infectious: It causes a chemical reaction in your body that lifts your mood. Not only that, but it also boosts your immune system, relieves stress, and helps others to see you in a positive light.
- Appreciate yourself rather than wait for others to appreciate you. Deciding that you are valuable and valued, and thinking positively about yourself, will slowly enable you to see yourself differently. Remembering your achievements can be an effective way to do this.
- Meditate to reset your mind. It can enable you to calmly organize your thoughts and shift the

focus of your problems. It can inspire creativity and inspiration, improve problem-solving skills, and allow you to get a good night's sleep. And it takes no more than 20 minutes daily (King, 2020).

- Spending time with your loved ones at least once a week prevents you from sliding into the downward cycle of depression and anxiety if you are that inclined (King, 2020). Spending time with friends and family will prevent you from locking yourself away from meaningful relationships that could help you. Visit a friend or take a long walk with one—you'll be so glad you did.
- Today, we're so attached to screens of one kind or another that it can be hard to tear ourselves away. But you must leave your house and visit someone else in theirs. Or walk your dog at the local park. Even just a few minutes in the fresh air can be invigorating and produce dividends throughout the day, increasing productivity and concentration. Going outside removes you from the stressful situations you cannot control, clearing your mind so that you can deal with them better.
- Turn off your phone or leave it behind. We've become so used to taking our phones

everywhere that we don't realize how insidious the tendency to check them constantly has become. This can increase your stress levels. It's important to unplug at some point. Do a hobby that doesn't involve technology at least once a week. Or read a book, preferably not on your phone.
- Exercise is essential to fuel emotional happiness. Even half an hour in the morning will ensure a happier day (King, 2020). Exercise allows more oxygen to reach your brain, reducing anxiety and depression. It also releases feel-good hormones that can naturally leave you feeling on top of the world.
- Learn a new skill. When we learn something new, our brain gets a rush of dopamine, a feel-good chemical. You'll also have more interests, which could improve your social life. A common interest is also great for developing new friendships. Take time to do whatever you've always wanted, whether it's an art class or learning to ski. This will improve your self-esteem too.
- Helping others is the ultimate feel-good—and helps to spread a positive attitude. Even small actions like giving an overloaded colleague a much-needed cup of tea can make a big

difference to them. Help others achieve their needs and desires. Be kind. You might be the one having a difficult day the next time, and they might help you.

WHO ARE YOU REALLY?

Before we can begin to love ourselves, we need to consider who we really are. The human psyche has three aspects: the false self (the delusionist), the ego, and the true self. So, who are all these personas hiding in plain sight?

The False Self

People create an artificial or delusional persona in their early childhood to protect themselves from re-experiencing trauma, shock, or stress in close relationships. As young children, we often believed that we had to comply with our parents' wishes and demands to be loved or tolerated—so we had to be false, in a sense, before we began to really live. This childhood mindset continues throughout our lives and is fostered by our education systems and even the careers we choose. Most of the time, we're simply putting on a compliant mask to be accepted or conform to what society, our boss, our spouse, or our community wants.

The Ego

The ego is a survival system we've evolved to protect ourselves. The main idea is that you've created this persona to reflect your opinions and views about who you might be. The biggest problem with ego is that our insecurities and self-doubts can influence it.

You'll likely have a poorly developed sense of self-worth if you have a fragile ego. Your thoughts will tend to be very self-destructive, and you'll continuously beat yourself up—metaphorically speaking, of course. Surprisingly, the converse—the big ego—is often little more than a psychological cover-up, where there's a lot of external self-validation to cover up deep, hidden insecurities. Those with big egos appear to think very highly of themselves and come across as self-confident and proud, with tremendous self-esteem.

The True Self

The true self has two aspects: a psychological one and a spiritual one. If you're searching for your true self, you're on a journey to discover your truth, even if doing so might make you uncomfortable before you're ready to embrace the freedom of knowing—and being—who you indeed are. You'll need to unmask your self-deluded thoughts and acknowledge your strengths, unresolved insecurities, and fears. As a result, you'll ultimately connect with your inner voice, which instinctively knows what's best for you and those around you.

Discovering your true self, psychologically speaking, can be described as developing a healthy ego. A quiet ego reflects healthy self-esteem, acknowledges its limitations, and is not afraid to be vulnerable. It doesn't become defensive when threatened and is firmly self-confident. It is less judgmental, more inclined to be rooted in reality, and has fewer boundaries.

From a spiritual point of view, the self or ego is an artificial construct. It consists of random pieces of information you have gathered during your lifetime. Being an artificial construct, if you don't protect it, it could break. The question is: Do you want it to?

The ego is all about itself—"I" predominates. It's all about your wants, needs, feelings, etc. The true self, however, can be summed up in one word, not "I" but "awareness." People who have quiet egos tend to look at everything as though they are outsiders.

VISUALIZE A POSITIVE RELATIONSHIP WITH YOUR CHILD

Picture you and your child in a few years. Ask yourself how your reactions now will affect your relationship in the future. We all want to have good, close relationships with our children, both now and in the future. It doesn't mean you need to give in to your child's demands or become a doormat. You must always treat your child with respect—as you would want them to treat you. Talk to your child the way you want your child to talk to you.

Think about the excellent relationship you want with your child, both now and when they are older or even adults. The foundation of a good relationship begins now. Keep this in mind when your anger threatens to overwhelm you. You don't want your children to be afraid of you or constantly mad at you. You don't want them to cut you out of their lives as soon as they leave home.

CREATING SOME "ME" TIME

Life can be so hectic sometimes that it's easy to become overwhelmed and stressed, which can fuel your anger and make you more likely to fly off the handle when faced with one of your triggers. We're all busy with work, raising children, family and household obligations, and more. It's therefore essential to make a point of setting aside some time—every day if possible—where you can be alone.

Practicing some meditation can help you find your own voice and enable you to understand who you are and what you want. It will make it easier to detach yourself from your emotions so that anger won't rule you.

LEARN TO SAY "NO"

If you tend to be a people pleaser—and many people do, especially women, as many of us are brought up that way—you'll probably identify with a comment someone left at the end of a YouTube video. The poster says she tends to be super-nice to someone for a long time, but one day she'll explode because she starts feeling that they're taking advantage of her good nature. She says she's becoming angry because she feels overwhelmed: In addition to holding down a full-time job and bringing up her daughter, she's running herself ragged doing things for others in her free time.

You might be a people pleaser if you can't seem to say "no," automatically agreeing to do whatever others ask of you, only to wish you hadn't just about immediately. You might also be inclined to put others' needs before your own. While the world needs a little kindness, you also need to ensure that your needs are met and that you have enough time to work, look after your family, and attend to everyday chores.

If you have difficulty setting boundaries with others, this is often because you're experiencing an internal struggle between your power as a human being and the need to foster a relationship with someone else. Besides saying "yes" when you'd far rather say "no," you might find yourself attacking the other person, saying "no" aggressively without considering their needs. This frequently happens with those closest to you, like family members, children, or spouses. Alternatively, you avoid the whole thing altogether by not providing a clear "yes" or "no" answer, prevaricating, or procrastinating. This can be highly negative, as you're not being honest with yourself or the other person.

It's essential to learn to say "no" in such a way that it empowers you while still maintaining your relationships with others. Constructively saying "no" enables you to have healthy relationships and gives others clarity on what to expect from you. You can take a little time if you need to evaluate your response first, but don't take too long and leave the other person hanging. Set a deadline by which you will provide an answer.

Make a list of your top three priorities to ensure that you say "yes" to the right things and put it where you'll nearly always see it. When someone asks you to do something, consider whether the task fits in with what you've decided will best use your energy and time. If not, then it's all right to say "no."

Tips for Saying "No" Effectively

- Be clear, confident, and consistent.
- Be short and to the point. There's no need to explain yourself at length.
- Have an anchor phrase. You can, for example, say things like: "I have a policy…," "I'd rather say no to you now than disappoint you later," or "I only support these charities."

TAKE GOOD CARE OF YOURSELF

Your child cannot take care of you. Self-love is when you put yourself before others—but it's never selfish. It's essential.

Prioritize Your Health

Get Enough Sleep

Regular sleep is vital for optimal health, and most adults should aim to get between seven and nine hours a night (Summer, 2022). While you sleep, your body repairs and rejuvenates itself, so getting a good night's rest is essential. Sleep has several other benefits:

- It improves your mood by elevating your energy levels the next day and reduces the likelihood of you becoming stressed. In fact, in 2013, Dutch children were regarded as the happiest in the world, mainly because they get plenty of sleep from infancy, as do parents, who might sleep for as long as 12 hours a night (Acosta, 2019).
- Quality sleep slows your heart rate and decreases blood pressure, enabling the heart and circulatory system to rest.
- Getting sufficient sleep regulates insulin and blood sugar levels in the body.
- It also boosts memory and cognitive functioning, improving concentration, problem-solving abilities, and effective decision-making.

- Growth hormones are produced during sleep, which enables development in children and young adults while restoring their bodies.
- When you sleep, your body produces cytokines, which support the immune system.
- Sleep produces the appetite suppressor leptin, helping to regulate body weight.

Exercise

Everyone knows that exercise is physically incredibly beneficial—it makes you stronger, fitter, and leaner. It may also reduce the likelihood of developing heart and lung diseases, high blood pressure, diabetes, obesity, cancer, and other health problems. As if that's not positive enough, exercise boosts your mental health. Being physically active releases endorphins and serotonin, which are natural mood improvers.

Endorphins are hormones your body releases when you are stressed or in pain. They are both natural painkillers and "feel-good" chemicals. Released during pleasurable activities, including exercise, they function as neurotransmitters—or messengers—in your body. When endorphins are attached to your brain's reward centers—or opioid receptors— dopamine, another "feel-good" chemical, is released. Your body produces more than 20 endorphins, which enhance your mental health (Cleveland Clinic, 2022). They ease depression, decrease stress and anxiety, increase confidence—which raises self-esteem—regulate your appetite, and even alleviate pain during childbirth. Serotonin helps stabilize your moods.

Exercise helps move blood to the brain, thereby improving your thought processes. It increases the size of the brain's memory part and expands the connections between the brain's nerve cells. Thirty minutes of moderate to intense physical activity should be sufficient for most adults to create these biological reactions (Health Direct, 2019).

Cultivate Good Eating Habits and Digestion

Stress, anxiety, depression, and emotions like anger take a heavy toll on the digestive system. Your esophagus goes into spasms, and your stomach produces less acid, giving you indigestion and heartburn. You could also suffer from diarrhea or constipation, bloating, and poor appetite. You might also develop gastric reflux, peptic ulcers, or irritable bowel syndrome (IBS).

One of the ways of calming your digestive system, apart from regulating your emotions and learning to deal with the life events that underpin them, is to implement strategies that support better digestion. Make sure to eat all meals. Eat three balanced meals every day. Chew your food well. Some sources say that each mouthful should be chewed as many as 32 times. It takes about 30 minutes for the stomach to inform the brain that it is full and you need to stop eating (Jain, 2017). Eat mindfully, eating the right amount of food without overeating or binge eating. Remember to drink plenty of water every day to avoid becoming constipated. You can also take a good probiotic to ensure the right balance of beneficial microbes in your gut.

But there's more to digestion than food. That might sound odd at first glance, but research increasingly shows that the brain and gut are connected. The digestive tract is densely packed with over 100 million neurons, the network of nerve cells that line it (Gerrie, 2020). Nicknamed the "second brain," this is, in fact, the enteric nervous system, which has more nerve cells than the spinal cord or peripheral nervous system. The gut has over 30 million neurotransmitters, signaling molecules more often associated with the brain in our heads. As much as 95% of the serotonin your body produces is created and stored in the gut (Gerrie, 2020).

The brain and gut "talk" to one another through the vagus nerve, a thick pathway of neurons running between the base of the brain and our gut. The gut is filled with hundreds of thousands of microbes and bacteria. Many of the former live in the mucus layer that lines the intestinal walls, placing them in direct contact with nerve and immune cells. Signals move back and forth, with 90% of the vagus nerve carrying information from the gut to the brain (Garrie, 2020).

What's happening in your digestive tract influences your moods biologically. Inflammation is often linked to mental illness, and many people suffering from depression and anxiety have been found to have inflammatory bowel disease. Stimulating the vagus nerve reduces inflammation and stress. Healthy bacteria in the gut encourage the brain to release natural calmatives like the neurotransmitter gamma-aminobutyric acid (GABA).

Quitting Smoking and Alcohol

It is obvious that part of looking after your physical health is to stop smoking—or at least cut down significantly if you are a heavy smoker. Consuming excessive amounts of alcohol is never a good idea—and it can inflame and aggravate your anger if you become aggressive after drinking alcoholic beverages.

ARE YOU FEEDING YOUR ANGER?

The body and mind are inextricably linked—to the point where even the foods we eat can profoundly influence the intensity of our angry emotions or belligerence. Trans fatty acids are conspicuously associated with greater aggression, while diets low in beneficial omega-3 fats have been linked to depression and antisocial behavior. The anger-regulating regions of the brain are affected by dropping serotonin levels. If that sounds fanciful, numerous scientific studies have verified these facts.

Low glucose levels in the blood may cause aggressive impulses if someone hasn't eaten. A three-month trial conducted at Australia's Deakin University found that 67 participants who had poor diets also struggled with moderate to severe depression (Amritha, 2021).

It makes sense at the biological level. Nutrient deficiencies can lead to various behavioral problems. Without the proper nutrients, the body cannot produce the so-called "happy hormones" required for clear thinking and a calm disposition. Some people might even exhibit irrational or dangerous behaviors because of their poor eating habits.

Modern Western medicine and natural Eastern and Ayurvedic medicine have found that certain foods are likely to aggravate an already angry disposition. These foods include tomatoes, brinjals (eggplants), cauliflowers, dried fruits and chips, chewing gum and candies, dairy products such as milk, yogurt, cheese, cold fruit, greasy foods, refined flour and sugar, and alcohol

(Amritha, 2021). It's essential to recognize that food affects different people in various ways. While eating tomatoes might make some individuals angrier, this might not be the case for everyone who eats tomatoes. Sodas, store-bought fruit juices, and coffee might also provoke mad people, as could eating bagels, agave nectar (a sugar substitute), cold meats, certain processed vegetable seeds, such as those of sunflowers or pumpkins, salted peanuts, margarine, french fries, canned foods, cereals, and wheat.

On the flip side, several foods may help you calm down if you are irritable. Bananas, for example, are rich in vitamins A, B, C, and B6, which all regulate the nervous system. Dark chocolate stimulates the release of endorphins and serotonin in the brain and reduces stress hormone levels. Walnuts contain nutrients for the brain. Other calming foods include baked potatoes, celery, spinach soup, and chamomile tea.

Dietary Recommendations for Anger Management

- Fish, poultry, eggs, and leafy green vegetables all help to increase dopamine production.
- Magnesium-rich foods like almonds, spinach, and pumpkin or sunflower seeds enable better quality, more restorative sleep.

- Limit your sugar intake. Eat more fruit and fewer candies.
- Include vitamin D-rich foods in your diets, such as fatty fish, egg yolks, and liver. Remember to spend plenty of time outside in the sun too.
- Eat more omega-3 fatty acids. You'll find them in fish, flaxseed, chia seeds, and walnuts.
- Adding colorful fruits and vegetables to your diet will boost your mood. It looks appetizing on the plate too!

CULTIVATING A POSITIVE MINDSET

Today, we are bombarded with "news." We watch it on our television sets before we go to work, listen to it on the car radio while driving, and consume more news in the evenings before we go to sleep. Some of us even subscribe to news apps to receive daily updates. As the media thrive on sensationalism, there tends to be more focus on "bad" news than "good." And our brains are wired to focus on the negative, so the news channels have us exactly where they want us.

If you're prone to anxiety and depression, it's no surprise that a steady diet of news is highly likely to make you feel worse. It can also fuel your anger if you have anger issues. Watching violent scenes, whether actual events or fictionalized, can make us think jumpy and lead to sleepless nights or troubling dreams. Yet, these conditions demand that we seek more certainty through having more information, so we're inclined to watch more news to find the solace we are looking for. We have the vague—and completely unfounded—idea that having enough information will help us wield more control over our circumstances. This makes us compulsively check news updates, making us feel worse.

Avoiding the news means that you don't need to have conversations focusing on the dreadful things happening in the world—or in your neighborhood—and disaster and chaos are not the focus of your social interactions with others. Not watching the news also gives you more time to do other, more positive things. Read a book, garden, find a new hobby, do a class, or visit a friend. You won't change the world by watching the news. And we live in such a highly connected world that you needn't worry about missing out on some important event. Somehow, you'll hear about it. It will be on social media, or a friend will mention it to you.

Choosing not to watch the news means your outlook automatically becomes more positive as you focus on the happier side of life rather than the grim news cycle. While you might find that some friends disapprove of your decision, you will meet others who embrace it, and your social circle will automatically become more positive.

If you still feel an all-encompassing need to consume news, there are a few things you can do to reduce your anxiety, depression, or anger. Ask yourself whether the information you're tuning into is helpful. If not, ditch it. Be selective of where you get your news and information from trusted sources. Set boundaries about how often you check news sites to ensure you don't become obsessive about watching the news. If people you interact with on social media spread information contributing to your discomfort, mute them or hide the posts from your feed.

HOW TO TRICK YOUR BRAIN INTO FEELING HAPPY

As we've learned more about how our brains work, we've discovered that fooling our brains into generating positive, happy states of mind is possible. But first, it's necessary to understand how the brain does this. The left prefrontal cortex is associated with more positive emotions; it will generate greater well-being if activated. In chronically stressed people, the brain initiates the release of cortisol, which effectively moderates the hippocampus, the part of the brain that produces visual-spatial memory, together with memory for context and setting. Such people eventually exhibit a reduced ability to form new memories. As the brain changes, so does the mind.

These changes can be either temporary or permanent. When changes are temporary, the flow of different neurochemicals will vary. For instance, people who consciously practice gratitude get higher inflows of reward transmitters, such as dopamine. It was also found that the reward centers in the brain light up when young couples who are romantically involved see photographs of their partners.

The mind can change the brain forever because what flows through the mind reshapes the brain. Busy regions of the brain start making new connections to one another. Depending on what's being activated, certain parts of the brain become physically larger.

You can therefore use the brain to change your mind for the better. The brain is continuously changing and remodeling itself—this is known as neuroplasticity. The key to changing it is to change what you are paying attention to purposefully. If you constantly focus on your resentments and regrets, your brain's physical structure will reflect those thoughts and feelings. But if you focus on things you are grateful for or life's blessings, you build up vastly different neural pathways in your brain.

The problem is that most people need to improve at managing their attention. We are constantly bombarded with new stimuli that our brains haven't experienced before. So, it's crucial that we focus on controlling our attention by cultivating mindfulness and gratitude. It's not enough to enjoy positive experiences, however. We need to hold onto them longer to ensure that they become welded into our brains.

If you have a positive experience that makes you feel good, like a good day at work or seeing a field of wildflowers in bloom, you need to hold onto the encounter for as long as possible. Savor it. Allow it to sink into you, using techniques such as visualization or prayer.

This is key to dealing with anger: You can train your brain to be positive, calm, and relaxed. Every emotion increases in intensity when we express it repeatedly. Focus on the things you're grateful for—like being a parent. Concentrate on your passions, excitement, and love. When you do this, these emotions will become stronger than negative emotions, like anger. When your personality is upbeat, you will see that you won't respond angrily the next time something upsets you.

KEYS TO GOOD ANGER MANAGEMENT

Our ego insists that we are right—no matter what. Although we might say that we are open to learning new things and developing fresh understandings of other people and situations, this belief goes out the window when we get into an argument. We start feeling that people are attacking who we are at our core rather than the ideas or opinions we may have. We are not our ideas.

It's also essential to learn not to take things personally. We sometimes get angry because we've taken something too personally. If someone we don't know well says something we don't like, we get mad, although the comment may not be directed at us at all. It's good to remember that when people say mean things and lash out, it's not about you but about them.

Another valuable aspect of anger management is learning when to let things go. We all want things to go our way—and we get upset when they don't. Until we can let go of our need to control situations or people, we will have difficulty reining our anger.

Avoid using strong and extreme language—words such as "never," "always," and "I can't stand it." Our terms drive intense feelings and make the anger even bigger.

We have very few actual "needs." Most of our demands boil down to things we want or desire.

Become aware of what's going on in your body. You might respond angrily or snap at someone for the reason that has nothing to do with their behavior—or yours—but rather concerns your own physical state. You might be hungry, tired, or stressed out, and that makes you lash out. Even getting too hot might increase your irritability. You then try to find a reason for the feelings, assuming that something has sparked them. It's vital to become mindful of what's going on in your physical body.

Learn how to express yourself clearly. For example, if your wife wants to have a conversation you know might be confrontational, but you are starving, tell her that you are hungry and suggest something to eat before that discussion. If you and your spouse are arguing because you're both tired, go to sleep. The situation might have resolved itself by morning, failing which you'll be better able to talk about it rationally. The more self-aware you become, the easier it will be to explain your physical state and feelings to others accurately. You may be feeling anxious. You could say to the person you are interacting with, "Look, I'm feeling a little anxious right now, and it's making me agitated and a bit annoyed. It's probably more to do with me than you, but perhaps we can have this conversation later?" Practice makes perfect. As you get into the habit of explaining accurately to others how you feel, the easier it will become.

PARENTS AS ROLE MODELS

As you embark on a self-care regimen and begin being kind to yourself, you will likely find your children following suit. As parents, we are role models and set examples for our children. Your efforts will encourage your children to accept themselves, forgive others, and be independently minded. They will know that they are always moving towards becoming a better person and be open to learning new things.

DESTIGMATIZING ANGER SO WE CAN TRULY ADDRESS THE PROBLEM

"You will not be punished for your anger, you will be punished by your anger."

— BUDDHA

How did you feel when you read the anecdotes I began the introduction with? It's my hope that you felt less alone and began to see that your anger isn't something to beat yourself up about, but something that you can learn to manage.

Remember the story about the father who was worried about the impact of his anger on his relationship with his daughters? He admitted that his outbursts were getting more violent and that this was troubling him.

That's a remarkably brave thing to admit, and it's a sign that this dad is on the way to overcoming his anger. Because when you realize that you're having an impact on those around you and you start taking responsibility for that, you're already taking the first step toward dealing with the problem.

That father was brave to admit what he did, and he probably doesn't realize the positive effect his words will have on others. When we share our experiences, we reduce the stigma attached to them so we can really deal with the problem without clouding it in shame, and we show other people that they're not alone and help is within their reach.

Without needing to divulge anywhere near as much detail as this man, you have an opportunity to do the same thing now.

By leaving a review of this book on Amazon, you'll show other parents that they're not the only ones fighting the anger battle... and you'll show them exactly where they can get the help they're looking for.

Simply by letting other readers know how this book has helped you and what they'll find inside it, you can help reduce the stigma associated with anger, and guide others toward a safe space where they can understand and address their issues.

Thank you so much for your support. When you're troubled by your anger, you often feel like you're the only one... And when you understand that you're not,  dealing with the problem becomes a whole lot easier.

Scan the QR code for a quick review!

4

BECOMING A PEACEFUL PARENT

> *A hot-tempered person stirs up conflict, but the one who is patient calms a quarrel.*
>
> — PROVERBS 15:18

If you know your triggers and change your perception, you can become a more peaceful parent. When conflicts arise, it's crucial to remember that anger often occurs when someone's desires and expectations aren't met. The only way to avoid falling into this trap is to be happy with what we have and to have fewer expectations of others.

Unrealistic expectations can frustrate and infuriate your children, and your own anger might intensify this with them. When parenting teens, it's essential to remind yourself that your children are growing up. This is the age when they explore the world to figure things out for themselves. They may not do everything you say. At this life stage, it's less about whom you want them to become and more about safeguarding them by ensuring they can learn, work, play, and socialize in a secure environment.

As I mentioned in chapter 2, while you may be very annoyed when your two-year-old throws an epic temper tantrum in front of your friends at the mall, understanding children's developmental stages will also help you manage your anger.

It can also be helpful to appreciate the difference between how you believe things should be (an expectation) and how they really are. This will help mitigate a lot of anger triggers. The key is to let go of your desires and accept the situation as it is, not as you would like it to be. Let's take road rage as an example. You might get angry when people drive too quickly or too slowly, or when the road design seems poor and illogical. Although you want everyone to drive smarter, you get annoyed because you're too attached to your idea of the "perfect driver."

It's helpful to realize that we rarely control what happens to us; nothing outside us is under our command. We only have control over our words and thoughts. While events may trigger unhealthy emotions, it is necessary for angry people to process these events in their minds.

BE PREPARED: WHAT TO EXPECT FROM YOUR KIDS

It is vital for parents to understand what to expect during their children's key development stages. Suppose your expectations are not closely aligned with your child's development path (where they will want more independence than ever, and you will need to initiate more push-back rules). In that case, you and your children will experience a lot of conflicts. However, the relationship is not static: As they get more independent, they will push back more. You can and should correct your children where necessary, but you also need to ensure that your expectations of them are realistic.

This means that if your 12-year-old leaves the kitchen looking like a war zone after baking chocolate cookies, you won't be mad at her. You realize that, at age 12, she is not yet a master of organization.

Erik Erikson, a psychoanalyst and professor at Harvard University, established the theory of human development. His model includes eight stages of psychosocial growth. In this chapter, I will list the key characteristics for each stage, together with tips for parents. I will cover the first five of Erikson's stages: 0–18 years, as these are the most important for human development.

FIVE STAGES OF HUMAN DEVELOPMENT

Stage 1: Birth to 18 Months

Key characteristics

During infancy, your child is entirely dependent on you. The act of crying when they are miserable and unhappy is designed to get your attention as a parent.

Tips for parents:

- Do not overlook your baby's needs for love and security.
- From both your voice and unique scent, your baby will learn to recognize that you are the person who feeds them and comforts them the most.
- You are the source of their happiness.
- Their crying is also an invitation for you to build a relationship with them. Whatever interaction you have with them, from changing diapers to burping—or simply holding your

baby—helps to deepen this relationship. This is crucial as it lays the foundation for future parenting.
- It's essential that parents be reliable and consistent. If they are not, then children will find the world an anxious, frightening place, and they will view it with mistrust. Children like this may develop behavioral problems later in life.
- Some studies show that anger-prone parents tend to give less care and love to their offspring, whose needs may not be adequately met at this stage of their lives.

Stage 2: 18 Months to 3 Years

Key Characteristics

As we all know, toddlers generally do not want or like to be controlled–and often make this blatantly obvious. They want to have autonomy and like to have their own way. They want to have their parents' undivided focus and to be the center of attention. This is also the age when children start exploring their world as they begin crawling and walking.

Tips for Parents:

- Be prepared to say "no" on numerous occasions. Toddlers will test the boundaries constantly, seeing how far they can go.
- One way of getting them to feel that they are making their own decisions is to ask them what sleeve they would like to put on first instead of asking them if they want to dress themselves.
- At this stage of childhood development, it is essential for parents to both allow and encourage their children to explore while providing them with guidance and ensuring that they are always protected.
- Children who are not allowed to assert themselves at this stage may well develop feelings of inadequacy and self-doubt, which can color the rest of their childhood—and even their teen and adult years.
- It's a crucial time for you to build on the relationship you founded with the child during infancy. Remember to spend plenty of time with your children so that your relationship can grow.

Stage 3: 3 to 5 Years

Key Characteristics

At this stage, children begin to interact socially by playing with others. They will usually take the initiative.

Tips for Parents:

- At this stage of their lives, kids ask an awful lot of questions—like "Why?" Be patient and give them age-appropriate answers or encourage them to find out more.
- Support them once they have made a decision.
- Allow them some degree of autonomy.
- Remember that, at this life stage, you are your child's idol.
- Too much criticism and excessively controlling behavior could cause children to lack ambition later in life or feel guilty for no reason.

Stage 4: 5 to 12 Years

Key Characteristics

Children at this age tend to compare themselves with others. They will work hard to reach their goals if they receive positive feedback from caregivers, teachers, and other authority figures. However, if feedback is negative, they may develop an inferiority complex.

Tips for Parents:

- Look for areas in which your children naturally shine. It can be sports, creative arts, academic achievement, or the ability to make good friends.
- At this stage, their teachers will be their idols.
- Bear in mind that this is when bullying by other children—or even adults—may start, so be watchful for signs that your child is being bullied—or is bullying others.

Stage 5: 12 to 18 Years

The teenage years can be divided into two categories, young teens (12–14 years old) and adolescents (15–18 years old) (Centers for Disease Control and Prevention, 2019).

Young teens are faced with an array of physical, mental, emotional, and social changes. As puberty arrives, hormones change, and your children's bodies mature into adulthood. These changes can lead to concerns about body image and self-consciousness. There may also be peer pressure to start experimenting with smoking, alcohol, or drugs or having sex. Eating disorders, depression, and family problems can plague some teens.

Adolescents whose bodies have matured (girls will grow faster than boys) might have weight, size, or shape issues. Girls especially may develop eating disorders. Besides having relationships with their peers, your teens may have relationships with other people, including adults, as they create a clearer sense of their uniqueness. It is a crucial time to prepare them for independence, as they may start working or go to college once they leave school.

Key Characteristics

This is when your child's sense of self develops and matures. They become more conscious of their appearance and body image. They frequently examine their beliefs, goals, and values. They may push back at parents and other authority figures to test their boundaries. They may even rebel.

Teens have an increased desire for independence, which may find expression in rebellious behaviors, like skipping school, breaking curfew, or sneaking out to meet a boyfriend or girlfriend. While this may be a cause for concern to adults, it is perfectly normal for teenagers to test the boundaries and extend their social interactions in preparation for adulthood.

Teenagers are often incredibly self-centered, and it's challenging to see things from another person's perspective. This is in part due to their still-developing brains. Adolescents may come across as being self-centered, focusing mainly on their own needs without considering those of others.

Despite this, their self-awareness tends to be unstable. Their interests, values, and sense of personal identity are constantly changing, depending on their peer group and other social influences. Because of this, as well as the physical changes they are undergoing, adolescents may question their place in the world.

When children reach adolescence, they might be more interested in developing relationships and more conscious of their sexuality. They should be more independent and have more capacity for caring, sharing, and developing close relationships with others. Their peer group and friends may become more important to them than their families during this time. They may be uncertain as to where they fit in socially.

Teens also experience intense emotions that change quickly. A teenager can easily be on top of the world one day and down in the dumps the next. This is particularly obvious in young adolescents. This mercurial behavior is exacerbated by stress. If these fluctuating emotions do not impair your child's functioning at home or school, it's nothing to worry about.

Tips for Parents:

- Be honest and direct when discussing subjects like smoking, drinking, drugs, and sex.
- Refrain from pressuring your teenagers to conform to your values or beliefs, or they might become confused.
- Take time to meet and get to know your children's friends and show an interest in their life at school too.
- Due to changes to the brain structure and hormonal changes, your child's emotions may shift very quickly. Social situations and interactions such as school and friendships could exacerbate this.
- Encourage your teens to make their own choices but guide them to make healthy decisions.
- Respect and consider your teenagers' thoughts and feelings. Make sure that they know you are listening to them.
- Relationships with their peers take precedence over their parents.

- Be clear about goals and expectations—things like getting good grades, keeping clean, and showing respect. Your teens should decide how they wish to implement these goals.
- Encourage your teens to become involved in volunteer and charity activities.
- Help them be responsible when using social media and ensure they know the potential pitfalls and dangers.
- Talk about responsibilities at work if your teens begin working, even on a part-time or casual basis.
- Help your teens plan ahead.
- Respect their privacy.

DO NOT BE AN EMOTIONAL ENSLAVED PERSON

Remember never to be enslaved by your own emotions—or those of another person. Bear in mind that emotions come and go. As such, it's vital that they don't rule you or dominate your life. Children or spouses don't make us angry; anger is something that happens within us.

According to Sadhguru, we have often decided what we like and don't like and which people we like—or don't like (Sadhguru, 2018). We've set our minds on whom we will cooperate with and whom we won't. This means that we have made a value judgment as to what —or who—is good and what—or who—is terrible. These attitudes are very polarizing for society.

Believing that we are "good" and everyone else is "bad" means that we have permitted ourselves to destroy those whom we have labeled as "bad." You might decide that people who aren't like you are "bad." This means that you have decided what goodness is.

It is our choice as individuals to decide who we are and how we will respond to a specific circumstance or event. We should not give our power over to others, allowing them to make us angry, unhappy, joyful, and so on. If someone else can determine how you feel at any given moment, haven't you allowed them to enslave you? External circumstances are often beyond our control, but our reaction to them is our choice. You may feel that you cannot work with certain types of people. But no one is perfect. If you think you are doing something significant, you must learn to collaborate with people you don't like.

PARENTING IMPERFECT

It's important to remember that you and your children are learning as you go along. Don't be afraid to make mistakes. Scrap the notion that you need to do everything exactly right. You cannot control or mastermind everything. Even if parents were perfect, children would make foolish decisions. You might struggle to be a good parent, and your children will still make wise choices. If you become angry in your parenthood journey, remember that you can use your anger to grow as a person—and improve your relationship with your child.

Be careful not to over-parent, as this prevents free play. Children won't learn to define a problem, find a solution, and solve the problem by themselves. Children are given to us for a season. They will eventually become independent people in their own right. We must equip them for adulthood.

Your relationship with your child is a two-way street. Even though you are a parent, your kids could still teach you a thing or two. Your child might enable you to see the wonder in small things—something that we easily overlook in our busy modern lives. Stop to look at a rainbow or spend time exploring a patch of wildflowers. You might also make new friends through your children, especially if they are extroverts.

Younger children tend to let it all hang out when expressing their emotions. This means that it's crucial to provide emotional support when your toddler is upset, or your ten-year-old has a bad day at school. It's essential to help them talk through what happened so that they can process it.

It means that we need to regulate our emotions so that we can be their sheltered place, their oasis of calm where they can go when storms hit. If you find yourself getting frustrated by your child's behavior when they are annoyed, sad, or upset, it's essential to learn to be patient, curb your temper, and find other, more constructive ways to deal with your feelings.

PUT YOURSELF IN YOUR KID'S SHOES

If we're having difficulties with someone who has done something we don't like, and they refuse to acknowledge our feelings, we might say something like, "Well, how would you feel if I did this to you?" By doing this, you've effectively suggested that they put themselves in your shoes. This tends to change the conversation, as people suddenly realize why you're so upset or angry with them—and that you're not being unreasonable.

In the same way, we need to put ourselves in our kids' shoes. They are not adults—and they cannot possibly see the world the same way we would, as they are still developing, exploring the world, and haven't had all the life experiences that we have. They're also from the next generation—and the world is changing so fast that they might well have different experiences to the ones you did when you were growing up.

You need to try to see the world from your children's perspective, attempting to see it the way they do, and consider how you would react to it if you were their age. Putting yourself in your children's shoes helps you relate to children of all ages, including teens and young adults. Your teenage daughter might decide she doesn't want to come down to dinner, yell at you when you call her, and perhaps even slam her bedroom door to emphasize the point. This might evoke a knee-jerk reaction in you, where you, in turn, lose your cool, yell back, take away privileges, or even ground her. Instead, think back to when you were that age. She could be facing some social crisis that feels like the end of the world. You remember what that was like.

Looking at life from your child's perspective can significantly benefit your relationship because you can come to the situation from a place of kindness and understanding rather than frustration and anger. Consider that your child's behavior is likely appropriate for their stage of development. Some forms of misbehavior might be sparked by them trying to cope with the experiences, feelings, and adult rules they face all day. The next time you are angry at your child, ask yourself how you would have reacted at that age. Their behavior will likely make more sense and help you handle the situation more positively and effectively. This also allows you to empathize with your child.

WHY DO MY CHILDREN ONLY LISTEN WHEN I YELL?

Some parents believe that the only way to get their children to listen to them—or to respond positively to instructions—is to express themselves angrily, yelling or shouting at their offspring. But trying to force cooperation in this way often has the unintended effect of kids tuning out, ignoring you, and doing exactly what they want. Sometimes you want to start yelling when you calmly ask your child to do something repeatedly, and they ignore the request.

Did you know that people can train one another to react in specific ways, pretty much in the same way as you teach your pet to respond to your commands? If you shout and yell all the time, you ultimately train your children only to pay attention when you are loud and angry. If you speak to them calmly, they seem to have no regard for the consequences of disobeying or ignoring you.

It's recommended that you move the stronger instruction up the queue so you don't wait until you fume because you can't get their cooperation. Just like we train kids to respond to us when we yell and shout, we can train them to respond when we first make a calm request.

It's important to remember that yelling and shouting do not qualify as disciplining or punishing your child. Shouting is simply a psychological reinforcer that you mean business. This means that yelling can even increase your child's bad behavior. However, punishment or discipline is likely to curtail it. Clinical psychologist Lori Osborne explains, "It's generally been well-established that high-intensity parent-child interaction, whether negative or positive, reinforces the behavior. Yelling has the opposite effect of what parents want because even negative attention like shouting and screaming is the attention most kids crave" (Advocate Arora Health, 2013).

Criticism from a parent is extremely hurtful for a child —because it comes from someone close to them. If a stranger on the road shouts out that you're ugly, you can ignore it because it won't upset you much: After all, they don't know you. But when someone you trust and respect says the same thing, it hurts a great deal more.

Parents need to encourage their children to think about their actions' consequences rather than fight with them. She suggests that parents set up rewards or consequences for good and bad behavior. Positively reinforcing good behavior usually sends a much stronger message than yelling and shouting when teens misbehave.

DEALING WITH SIBLING RIVALRY

You might start to feel anxious when your children start rowing with one another. It's important to remember that sibling rivalry is a normal part of growing up and helps children develop emotionally and socially. It teaches children how to cooperate, resolve conflict constructively, and be responsible. It also increases their kindness and empathy.

There's a certain inevitability about sibling rivalry, however. Your oldest child was once the center of attention—until you brought home their baby brother or sister. Now they have to wait in line while the baby's needs are dealt with. Later, the children will want to play with the same toys or get tired of being bossed around. Children misbehave because they don't necessarily like the new person you brought home and often see them as competition for your time, attention, and affection.

Sibling rivalry may begin when a child feels they are not being recognized as a separate, unique person in the household and as being special to their parents. Children need to feel that they are loved equally and fairly treated. Sibling rivalry happens when one child is afraid that other siblings may be treated better.

Tips for Handling Sibling Rivalry

- Your children should have some belongings that are theirs alone and shouldn't need to share everything.
- Praise and focus on both—or all, if you have more than two—your children's good points, such as teamwork, persistence, or kindness. Siblings learn to support one another rather than compete for your attention.
- Give each child at least 10–15 minutes of kid-centered, intentional attention daily (Positive Parenting Solutions, 2009). This means that they are in control—they decide what you will do, and you need to enter into the spirit of the thing, whether it's a doll's tea party, doing a puzzle, or running alongside while they ride their bike.
- Take each of your children out alone on a mom (or dad) and one child outing or adventure.

Choose what you will do and have the child who enjoyed the outing bring something home for the other. This helps them understand that while they may do some activities together or as a family, they might also do other things alone or with you or your spouse. This enables them to see themselves as different individuals and understand the boundaries of others around them.

- Encourage direct communication rather than flying off the handle when one child exhibits antisocial behavior, like taking things from the other without asking first. Teach children to take turns when playing with their favorite toys and encourage them to use appropriate language with "I feel" statements. Teach them techniques to cool down after a fight, such as counting to ten, walking away, etc.
- Let them fight but be careful to stay out of it. Ignore it as much as possible to allow them to work things out themselves. If things start escalating, step in, being careful to listen to each child's version of what happened and get them to come up with solutions.
- If no agreement can be reached, then decide what happens. For example, tell children you will put the game away unless they take turns.

- Ensure that they know that you value empathy, generosity, kindness, and encouragement, and urge them to behave like this towards one another.
- Step back when one child is upset and allow the other to comfort them.
- Avoid saying "you" to both children when you scold or praise them, as they are two individual people.
- Avoid saying things like: "Why can't you keep your room tidy as your sister does?" Constantly comparing your children to one another in this fashion is not conducive to fostering the behavioral change you want, which will help them later in life.
- Never go to bed angry. Ensure that conflicts are resolved before bedtime.

COPING WITH TANTRUMS AND MELTDOWNS

Tantrums and meltdowns can be wearying, irritating, and even embarrassing if they happen in a public place like a supermarket aisle or a park packed to capacity on a sweltering summer day. Sometimes you're at a loss as to why your child is so upset.

Children develop exponentially from birth until about seven years of age. This means that you're bound to see tremendous swings in their moods and emotions. They're learning how to feel and express their feelings positively. Our job as parents is to empathize with our children, letting them know that their feelings are real and that they matter.

Children need to express their emotions. Smacking a crying child might make them feel it's not okay to cry when sad. After all, crying helps us process our feelings, and many of us feel better after a good cry. If your child's crying triggers your anger, take a step back. Acknowledge your anger, breathe, and empathize with your child: "Hey, that must have upset you. How about a hug?"

The biggest challenge for you as a parent caught in the storm of a child's tantrum is to force yourself to regulate your own emotions. Children will mirror the stress and feelings of the adults around them. When you are calm, you can respond with new insight, compassion, and patience toward them. It's essential to model the behaviors you're trying to teach your children. If you react negatively to emotions that make you feel uncomfortable or that trigger you, such as anger or tears, then all you do is teach your children to suppress them.

Never give in to your child's demands if they use the attention generated by a tantrum to get their way. They might have seen another child do this—and get away with it—so they try it too. Or they may have discovered they can get their way by throwing tantrums with their parents or other adults around them. If you don't reward bad behavior, it will stop on its own.

Put your ego aside and consider everything that might have led to the tantrum. When things are calm again, discuss how your child can better express themselves and their feelings. Point out that you'll understand things better if they are calm and explain what they need. Give your child your full attention when they are speaking, so they don't feel the need to resort to tantrums.

Nearly always, children are just trying to get their needs met. There is nothing personal or intentionally hurtful about their behavior. Your child needs your energy, concern, and presence when they are upset and having a meltdown. Doing so will encourage them to express their emotions more appropriately. However, when their anger provokes you to a reaction, then all you do is teach them to repress their feelings. This is not the same as controlling your emotions without outside intervention.

WHAT TO DO WHEN YOUR CHILD IS ANGRY: HINTS AND TIPS

A three-year-old child throws her toys around the room, stamps her feet, and lies down on the ground when she hears the word "no." She also hits the person who says it and tends to scream a lot. Her babysitter says the child has a short temper. After looking after this little girl for a week, the babysitter is at the end of her tether.

The above scenario is particularly prevalent in children who have trouble expressing their emotions, and it can be a very frightening experience for parents and other caregivers. The child will often be remorseful once they have calmed down or exhausted themselves.

So, what do you do when your child throws a scary temper tantrum like this, lashing out physically at you or others?

While it's tempting to dismiss the episode as attention-getting or manipulative, it's important to remember that children who do this lack the ability to express their anger and frustration constructively. They need help to talk it through and arrive at a solution.

The first thing to understand is that all behavior is a form of communication. A child who does this is very distressed. This is compounded by the fact that they may not have the language skills to express their feelings verbally. They may also have difficulty with impulse control or problem-solving. At this point, how you react—or don't—to the meltdown will determine whether they continue to respond to stress in the same way or learn to handle their emotions better.

Your response to a tantrum also depends on how severe it is. Non-violent tantrums should be ignored as far as possible, as even negative attention—like asking the child to stop doing something—can be interpreted as encouragement by the child. However, this is not recommended when the child is physically lashing out, as this can endanger them and others. When this happens, move the child to a safe environment where they cannot access you or anything else that may have good associations.

Three-year-old children naturally exhibit this type of behavior, however, and it should be considered perfectly normal. Young children are impulsive, demanding, and highly interactive. Don't give in to them. Sit with the child while they express these intense emotions. Be kind, compassionate, and caring so you model the correct behavior to them. When they are calm, talk about gentle hands and feet that don't hurt others.

Here are some quick tips as to how to respond when a child throws a dangerous tantrum:

- It's vital that you stay calm in the middle of the storm. Don't shout, as this will probably make things worse. You also have less chance of getting them to hear you. Keep your own emotions under control. This teaches the child the value of stillness.
- Safety is also essential. Remove whatever can be removed during the tantrum to ensure no one gets hurt physically. Keep the child safe by holding them and gently rocking them until they calm down. Then talk about what happened, suggesting better ways to express their feelings once they are fully ready. Remember to reward them when they begin to self-regulate without adult intervention.
- Don't give in. If the tantrum occurred because you said "no," then don't agree with what the child wants to make it stop.
- You can also let them throw a tantrum but ignore it. When they're done, praise their good behavior. Have them clean up the toys they threw around during the tantrum. Perhaps you can help. When they hit you, calmly grab their arms to stop them from doing this, but don't

say anything about it. Let go as soon as they stop trying to hit you.
- Once they've calmed down, praise them for getting it together. When they start expressing their feelings verbally, calmly or try to reach an agreement with you, commend them for their efforts.
- Practice problem-solving with your children. When your child is not upset, help them talk about their emotions and suggest solutions to potential conflicts before they get out of control. Ask them how they feel and suggest that they come up with ideas if you disagree.
- Some sources suggest that if children are younger than seven or eight years old, you can implement a "time-out" for non-violent outbursts (Child Mind Institute, n.d.). This involves having the child sit on their own for a few minutes in a room from which all pleasurable items have been removed. After the child has calmed down, they must sit in a "time-out" chair.
- But another, more contemporary take on managing furious and upset children is to opt for a "time-in" approach. As with the "time-out" approach, the caregiver removes the child from the situation but then spends time with them

instead of leaving them alone, helping them to release their angry emotions safely and bringing the problem under control. It's essential to show empathy and understanding for how the child feels during the "time-in." This is often sufficient to calm down a fraught child. Research has found that parents who typically value and accept their children's emotions have children who feel secure, have lower anxiety, and have better social interactions with their peers.

- Another alternative is a feeling break. Inappropriate behavior arises from over-stimulation, hunger, tiredness, or just the inability of your youngster to express their emotions. Take a short break (about four minutes) and remove your child from the activity or other children—or even yourself if necessary. Talk to your child about their emotions and briefly remove yourself from them, remembering to reassure them that you will be there when they're feeling more relaxed and that you are close by. If it's close to mealtime, give them a snack, as hunger may be causing the meltdown.
- Remove yourself from the area for older children, so you are not at risk. If the situation

persists, you may need to call emergency services to ensure everyone's safety.
- You could implement a reward system for appropriate behavior, such as points or tokens towards something your child wants.
- Avoid triggers. Most children who have meltdowns tend to have them at specific times of day—homework time, bedtime, the end of playtime, and so on. They won't like having to stop doing something they enjoy or do something they don't like. Ways to avoid triggering your child include giving time warnings (e.g., "We're going in ten minutes") or breaking down tasks into small steps, like putting on their shoes before leaving. You can prepare a child for a potentially uncomfortable situation, reminding them to ask to be excused from the table before they slip out of their chairs, for example.
- If the vicious meltdowns are happening so frequently that they disrupt your family life, you may need professional help. Trained professionals can assist you with behavioral therapies and techniques to help you—and your children—manage their behavior.

When It's More Than a Tantrum

If tantrums and meltdowns frequently occur, more intensely, or past the age when children can be expected to behave in this way, there could be an underlying problem that needs treatment. Some possible reasons for ongoing aggressive behavior include the following:

- Children with ADHD are easily frustrated.
- Anxious children hide their worries but lash out when they are under pressure. They may be fine at school but lose it at home.
- An undiagnosed learning disability may cause the child to act out at school or when doing homework because the schoolwork may be too difficult for them.
- Some children are easily overwhelmed by sensory information. They don't like noise, crowds, or "scratchy" clothes and may become anxious, uncomfortable, or overwhelmed. The cause of the meltdowns may be a mystery to you.
- Autistic children across the spectrum become aggressive and throw tantrums when faced with change or frustration. They may have sensory issues too.

It's essential to get a correct diagnosis when your child continues to be aggressive and throw violent tantrums for no apparent reason. Once diagnosed, you may be referred to a specialist for further treatment. Treatments may include certain medications or learning to use safe holds on your children, so they cannot injure you or themselves. Children may sometimes need to spend time in a residential treatment facility. Alternatively, the child may live at home but attend a special needs school.

If you have an explosive child, take the time to learn how to deal with them behaviorally, as this could make all the difference to them, you, and your family life. Being confident, calm, and consistent will help your children develop skills to regulate their behavior.

Remember that sometimes children will press your buttons just to get your attention—and they know exactly how to do this.

5

STAYING CALM WHEN YOUR CHILDREN PUSH YOUR BUTTONS

> *When angry, count to ten before you speak. If you are outraged, count to one hundred.*
>
> — THOMAS JEFFERSON

Even if you're doing everything right as a parent, you will occasionally lose your temper with your kids. Children are smart and quickly learn exactly how to push your buttons. However, your reaction is entirely under your control. It's up to you to discipline yourself to handle anger properly. In this chapter, I will explain how to constructively voice your anger using ancient wisdom and techniques stretching back over 2,000 years.

EXPRESSING YOUR ANGER CONSTRUCTIVELY

It's important to remember that angry parents will produce angry children. We learn appropriate—or inappropriate—behaviors from our parents and other adults we interact with as we are growing up. In the previous chapter, I dealt with the destructive habit of yelling at your children. It's easier said than done, but before you start shouting, remember that yelling at your children will instill fear into them, which might cause them to suppress their emotions. When they grow up, they will likely be as angry as you are. Several case studies show that many children with anger issues come from families where the parents are also mad people. This is one of the root causes of those invisible triggers discussed in chapter 2.

As a parent, you must ensure that you are as calm and understanding as possible, as this will engender trust in your children. When dealing with teens especially, it's essential to talk to them as equals and adults instead of screaming at them as though they were small children. If treated like this, they might become resentful, sulky, or angry and won't cooperate. Remember that children react to the tone of your voice, not just the words you say.

One study published in 2013 stated that using screaming to discipline your teenager might exacerbate bad behavior. Researchers at the University of Pittsburgh found that harsh verbal discipline could be as psychologically damaging to a teen's developing personality as physical abuse. Considering nearly 1,000 children aged 13 and 14, together with their parents, researchers found that when parents used increased shouting to discipline 13-year-olds, this led to an increase in behavioral issues and depression in 14-year-olds (Advocate Arora Health, 2013).

Martin Teicher, an HMS associate professor of psychology at McLean Hospital, found that when children witness explosive expressions of anger, this can be pathogenic (Dougherty, 2022). It is difficult for people to see such raw and intense emotions, which can leave them emotionally scarred. Children's brains react by dialing down the impact of abusive words, images, and even physical pain. This means these sensory pathways become blunted and don't function as they should.

Physical punishment should likewise be avoided as far as possible because it can affect children even more negatively than yelling. The best way to get children to behave or listen without yelling or flying off the handle is for parents to set up consequences—for both bad and good behavior. Children then need to make choices and learn to live with the results.

How to Get Children to Listen Without Yelling

One way of doing this is to offer children a choice of two actions that are both acceptable to you when you ask them to do something. This means they will need to consider these options before the situation becomes a fight. This empowers children, as they believe that they are making decisions for themselves. If they refuse to choose one of the options you offer, you make a choice for them.

In some scenarios, especially for teens, one choice might have negative consequences if they refuse to listen. However, it's not a good idea to place too much emphasis on the negative outcome. Giving them options enables children to understand and experience the consequences of the actions they have chosen.

An excellent example of this—and I'm sure we've all heard this one—is when a toddler refuses to go to bed when it's bedtime. One of his parents will say, "Either you walk up to bed yourself, or I will carry you." In this case, the child will probably want to be carried, which is fine, and this avoids you having to start a war with them when they refuse to cooperate.

Here's a great story to illustrate the point. A mother of teenagers, frustrated with the endless battle to get her children to clean up their rooms, gave them this choice: "You can pick up your clothes and stuff from the floor, or I can do it for you. But you won't like it when I do it because I will leave those rooms spotless." The teens ignored their mother's request—and came home to find that their rooms were almost bare. Their mother had left them with a set of night clothes, their school uniforms, sports gear, and some pens and paper. Everything that had been on the floor or not put away was removed. They then earned these items back one at a time by proving that they could clean up after themselves daily and keep things tidy. Those kids sure listened to their mom after that!

Diverting Your Attention to Release Energy

If you shout or throw an adult tantrum, this harms you and the people around you. You need to learn how to divert your emotional energy in a peaceful and constructive way. Even if you feel a lot better after punching a wall, for instance, it still harms your health because your emotions will release a lot of toxins into your body. Remember that anger is an emotion that builds up and gets more intense and ultimately violent if you constantly give into it.

Because of this, you gradually change your personality whenever you get angry. You become angrier every time you succumb to your fury. The key to solving this problem is to focus on and generate good emotions. However, not releasing strong emotions correctly creates a vicious circle—an emotional dead end.

There are several ways to do this, but one of the key methods is to divert your attention, so your body will delay or ignore the signals that usually make you explode. Parents should adopt the ways that suit them and their lifestyles.

Hints and Tips

- Get active. You can release your anger auto-chemically, encouraging your body to release "feel-good" endorphins through exercise. For instance, you could drop down on the floor and do, say, 50 push-ups. At this point, the brain will start releasing endorphins, which override cortisol. If you do this often, you'll train your brain: It will automatically release endorphins to counter the inflaming effects of epinephrine and cortisol.
- Some other types of exercise you can do to facilitate this—and release your angry feelings—is to go to a gym equipped with punching

bags. Alternatively, go for a run and pound the sidewalk as fast as possible. You can also go for a long swim, as this also helps control your breathing, which physically reduces anger and rage.
- Doing your favorite things will often enable you to release strong emotions. Do artistic stuff like pottery, scrapbooking, drawing, or painting. Work on handcrafts like sewing or knitting, listen to your favorite music, go for a walk, spend time with a pet, or tickle a rubber band.
- Breathe. One way of controlling anger is deceptively simple. We all breathe. Picture a coil unwinding gradually as you breathe out through your stomach. Take slow breaths in and out. Then imagine yourself winding the coil and slowly letting it go. This calms you down. If necessary, do this several times until you feel calmer. You can also include the adage of counting to ten by breathing in and out as you count.
- Slide an elastic band onto your wrist when you feel angry and are tempted to start shouting. Flick yourself with it, and you'll find the need to yell reduces.

- Remind yourself that the angry feelings won't last. This will enable you to stop your negative responses when your blood starts to boil.
- Some people tend to burst into tears when they are outraged. This can release tension—and most people feel better after a good cry.
- Hugging someone can also defuse angry feelings.
- Some people find washing their faces or having a cold shower helpful.

But what happens when you can't leave the room or the situation is such that you don't have a few minutes to breathe? Or if your anger comes out of the blue, hitting so quickly that you forget every anger management technique you have learned?

THREE-STEP NPA ACTION FOR INSTANT RELEASE

This technique can be used by anyone, anywhere, and is an organic way to get past extreme anger when the blood rushes to your head. It is referred to as the Nod-Press-Ask (NPA) action.

The techniques I am about to explain are rooted in Taoism, which goes back around 2,300 years (Moeller, 2012). Most of you will probably be familiar with the

Taoism symbol of the yin/yang diagram in a black and white pattern. Through the ages, it has been the most important strain of Chinese thought after Confucianism. Taoism is one of the mainstream religions in east Asia today. Both Taoism and Confucianism share Chinese ideas and concepts that emphasize living in harmony with the Tao. This is the source of everything—and the ultimate principle underlying reality.

Taoism has contributed significantly to the development of Chinese Traditional Medicine (TCM). One of its founders, the ancient Chinese philosopher and writer Lao-tze, was Confucius' teacher (551-479 BC) (Wikipedia, 2022). Confucius is ranked 5th in Wikipedia's ranking of the 100 most influential people in history—after Muhammed, Isaac Newton, Jesus, and Gautama Buddha (Wikipedia Contributors, 2022).

Step 1

Nod Slowly when you feel that initial rush of anger.

This simple Taoist trick helps people process their anger and provides instant relief. The idea is that if you can nod, you can admit that everything in the world is ultimately acceptable.

Step 2

Press your anger valve—the CV 17 point (Larsen, 2016).

In TCM, the chest center acupuncture point (CV 17 point) is a crossing point for the lung, pericardium, and heart channels, which makes it a great place to open the chest (see diagram). This helps clear phlegm and congestion, resolve anxiety or panic attacks, calm heart palpitations, and relieve acid indigestion.

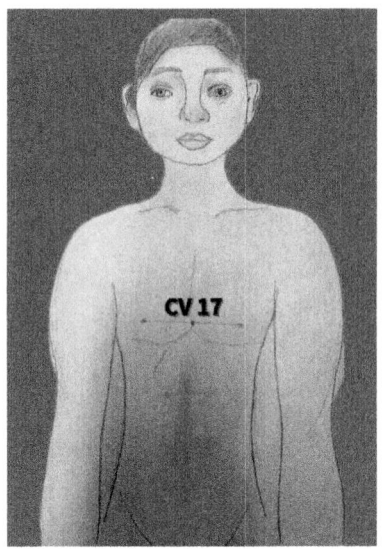

The ancient book *The Yellow Emperor's Classic of Medicine*, written more than 2,000 years ago, is one of Taoism's most important reference works. This ancient

Chinese medical text has been regarded as the premier authority on TCM for more than two millennia (Maoshing Ni, 1995). According to this text, the chest center point is a guard for the heart and a messenger of happiness and joy.

Acupuncture is an ancient Chinese treatment that has been systematically used for over 2,000 years and is now rapidly gaining ground as a Western alternative option (Liang and Wu, 2006). It is used as a complementary therapy for its positive effects in relieving pain and certain neurological conditions, including cancer, strokes, mood disorders, sleep disorders, and inflammation. Over the past 20 years, there has been a lot of research into the therapeutic benefits of using acupuncture as a medical treatment. Over 30,000 studies have been conducted in 60 countries, affirming the results from thousands of historic human and animal studies (Kopperman, n.d.).

Recommended by doctors and acupuncture professionals, CV 17 is a great self-help point to free the heart of tension while connecting to the heart as a whole. It is located in the middle of the line that connects the two nipples. For moms, the easiest way to find it is to follow your bra band into the center of your chest under your arm. When you look at the location of CV 17, you may notice that it matches the location of the heart chakra.

When open, this embraces our ability to open our hearts, allowing us to love deeply and completely.

To stimulate CV 17, use your 2nd or 3rd finger to press the point with a clockwise or counter-clockwise motion. Hold the point for a minute and repeat this a few times. Remember that your finger must press CV 17 with a bit of pressure. You may feel a little sore when you press it, but make sure you find it correctly. You can also take a breath while you stimulate the point.

Even if you are not feeling angry, you can do this. It is an excellent exercise while sitting in your car waiting at the traffic lights. You can add it to your bedtime routine, as it will promote better sleep and improve your health at no cost.

Step 3

Ask yourself whether your situation will bother you five months from now. If the answer is "no," you should let go of your anger. This step helps you realize that nothing is so important as to allow yourself to get angry when things don't go your way. The angry feelings will expire if you practice delaying or waiting before venting.

OTHER WAYS TO DEAL WITH ANGER CONSTRUCTIVELY

Use Positive Self-Talk

Positive self-talk may sound like nonsense, but behavioral psychologists have been recommending and endorsing it for decades. We all talk to ourselves in a manner of speaking—it's that "voice" in your head that only you hear. The good news is that you can decide how to respond to a given situation.

Consider past events. If you've faced a similar situation in the past, how did you defuse it successfully? What soothes you when you have an uncomfortable experience? Say something to yourself that helps you to stay in control: Tell yourself to breathe, slow down, or stop. Ask yourself whether this really matters or if it's important in the long run.

Having a tranquil mental picture to focus on when you start feeling triggered is another useful coping mechanism. Go to your favorite quiet place in your mind. Visualize it when you're anticipating a conflict situation with your child.

Tell yourself that you are empowered and that you can do this.

Take a Deep Breath

Stop and take a deep breath when you find yourself escalating, starting to yell, or losing control. This not only sends oxygen to your brain but also stops the flow of negativity and fury. Don't react reflexively. Think about what you want to say and respond actively.

Taking a deep breath will interrupt your automatic response. Deep breathing helps to reverse what happens biologically when you get angry. It signals to the body that everything is okay, reducing its fight-or-flight response.

Besides, doing this will give you time to consider what is going on and think about what you want to say. Your child might also notice that you've stopped reacting—and the extra minute might also give them time to reconsider their position too.

Breathing Techniques to Manage Anger

The following breathing technique will help to reduce the physical impact of anger on your body and takes only a few minutes. It lowers the heart rate and eases the mind by raising oxygen levels. This helps you focus on what is going on. Also known as 3-9-6, this technique restores calmness while reducing anger and frustration (Sources of Strength, n.d.).

While doing this exercise, take deep breaths, breathing from the belly rather than the chest. Breathe in deeply through your nose for three counts, hold your breath for nine counts, and then exhale through your mouth for six counts (Sources of Strength, n.d.). Before you begin, ensure that your stance or posture is as open as possible: uncross your feet, legs, and arms. Sit comfortably upright and let your gaze rest on anything in the room. If other people are with you, it's best not to look at them.

Then do the breathing exercise above, focusing on your breathing and counting. You will often calm down automatically when you're doing this, and whatever triggered you will also recede.

MEDITATION FOR LONG-TERM ANGER MANAGEMENT

Meditation concentrates your attention on something, whether it's a physical action like breathing or an external object, sound, or movement. Meditation doesn't empty the mind but trains it to focus, allowing the nervous system to balance itself, thereby calming you down naturally.

Resolving anger issues through meditation can help break the cycle by addressing the thoughts, feelings, and biological responses anger evokes. Meditation disrupts the fight-or-flight response, encouraging self-regulation. It literally quietens down the amygdala, shutting down the automatic stress reaction and slowing the release of stress hormones like adrenaline and cortisol. The brain has a natural capacity to change, transform, and grow. Meditation allows it to readjust its habitual responses and behavioral patterns.

Meditation as a tool for anger management can help to reduce the cycle of negative thoughts. It increases our awareness of our emotions so that we respond appropriately and less impulsively. It also increases our stress tolerance and ability to observe and remain detached.

Many studies have established that mindfulness, including meditation, reduces anger, aggression, and hostility. A 2015 study found that cortisol levels dropped among participants who meditated regularly (Peterson, 2021). Another study found that people who meditated remained emotionally calm when remembering events that had angered them, while non-meditating participants began feeling angry all over again.

Below are some meditations that may help mitigate your anger.

Being Led by Breath

Focus on your breathing rather than your thoughts and emotions. The soothing rhythm of breathing releases tension and anger, allowing you to connect with that part of yourself that isn't angry.

Inhale slowly and deeply while imagining a soothing white light filling your body. Hold your breath for two counts, gathering up the feelings of tension and anger (Peterson, 2021). Exhale slowly and completely, imagining the anger leaving your body as you do. Feel the stress leaving as your entire body relaxes.

Releasing Anger From Your Body

This meditation considers the physical sensations and tension in your body when you are angry or stressed. It allows you to release it consciously.

As you breathe, focus your attention on different parts of your body, one at a time, starting with your feet, then your legs, torso, neck, arms, hands, and fingers. Clench and relax each area as you inhale and exhale. Finally, imagine the anger draining from your body and away from you.

Being a Neutral Observer

Practice observing your thoughts and emotions, increasing your awareness of them without judgment. Notice whether diverting your thoughts in this way reduces your impulse to act out.

Choose something specific to focus on. It can be the sound and feeling of your breath or an actual object. Take note of sensory details like sounds, textures, nuances of color and shape, sensations in your body, and so on. When your mind wanders, what emotions do you feel? Stay with them and notice how your body responds. Resist any urge to stop or act on any of these emotions. Let them float out of your awareness as you turn your attention back to your breathing or the object you focus on. Continue shifting your focus from how you feel to the thing until you no longer wish to react to what triggered your anger.

Breathe Colors

Anger is red. In this meditation, visualizing colors helps shift your perspective so you can see the world and yourself in other shades.

Don't try to play down the way you feel. Imagine your body becoming saturated with red as you breathe. Notice the sensations in your body as you do this. Now picture your favorite colors, breathe them in, and allow them to dissipate the red. Exhale, feeling these delightful colors infusing the space around you. Please think of the happy, pleasant experiences they evoke and focus on them as you continue breathing in and out. Notice when angry thoughts and feelings start creeping in and see how this changes the colors you are seeing. Finally, take a deep breath as you imagine yourself bundling up the red anger. Breathe out, visualizing it leaving your body like an unwanted cloak, never to return. Then continue breathing in your contented color.

Boosting Self-Regulation

Self-regulation, self-control, or discipline is a trait everyone has, but it can be difficult to draw on it when we're blinded by anger. This meditation brings self-control to the forefront of your mind so that anger releases its hold on you.

1. Breathe in, thinking, "I am in control."
2. Breathe out, thinking, "I release my impulsive urges."

3. Breathe in, saying, "I know I am stronger than my anger."
4. Breathe out, saying, "I step out of my anger."
5. Breathe in, thinking, "I make conscious choices myself."
6. Breathe out, thinking, "I free myself from anger's clutches."
7. Breathe in, thinking, "I am in control."
8. Finally, breathe out.

Increasing Awareness and Curiosity

While anger is a natural human emotion, it limits us by threatening to take over our thoughts, physical sensations, and actions. You can enlarge your thoughts and feelings by approaching anger with curiosity to create more psychological balance.

First, allow yourself to feel the anger. Notice how it affects your mind and body. As you breathe, allow yourself to feel the anger but don't try to change it or react to it. Establish what you feel in your body, allowing it to exist and expand. Then consider the physical world around you. Let your gaze wander without settling on any single thing. Take in any sounds you hear, fragrances you smell, or lingering tastes in your mouth. Acknowledge them without doing anything about them. Finally, allow your thoughts and feelings to drift back to your angry state. Acknowledge how you feel.

Using Kindness to Deflect Anger

If we judge ourselves and others harshly, this makes it difficult to break free from an angry state. Acknowledging the good in someone else doesn't ignore the fact that they have wronged you but allows you to broaden your perspective, remembering that there's more to someone (including you) than their annoying behavior.

Start off by thinking about someone you have positive, kind feelings for. Allow yourself to consider them with warmth and tenderness. Mentally say to them, "May you be safe, healthy, happy, and at ease." Then, picture yourself and make the same wishes. Next, visualize the person who has made you angry and notice how your body changes in response. Feel the feelings and then ask yourself whether there is more to that person, including their strengths and other positive actions they may have done. I wish them safety, health, happiness, and ease.

6

DIFFUSING PARENTAL ANGER

> *Mindfulness is a way of befriending ourselves and our experiences.*
>
> — JON KABAT-ZINN

If your angry outbursts ambush you without warning, then this chapter will be very beneficial for you. In it, you will discover how to stay one step ahead of situations that typically trigger your anger. Living more mindfully is key. Listen to your anger rather than becoming a conduit for it.

Remember that anger management is a lengthy process and involves discovering how to practice mindfulness. You need to train yourself in it even when you are not angry. Ask the question: "Is getting angry making me happy or joyful? Is it improving my health?" If your answer is a resounding "no," you need to question why you allow your temper to get out of control.

If you constantly lose your temper with your children or lose control, it is essential to admit that you have a problem. Reflect on the triggers you encounter and your reactions to them, and consider ways to avoid getting angry when something triggers you.

A USEFUL TIP

To establish just how often you start feeling angry, you could practice the art of "hammering in a nail" in a manner of speaking. Carry a pocket diary around and draw a line on the date page indicating each time you find yourself becoming angry. You could also put a piece of paper on your fridge daily and mark it every time your anger stirs. It's a good idea to make this a habit so you remember to record your angry moments. This will enable you to become more aware of when you get mad and how often you feel this way. Because you have raised your awareness of what is happening, you will likely find it easier to control your reactions and subdue your anger.

EXPRESS YOURSELF IN A MINDFUL WAY

When it comes to your children, it is essential to explain to them what behaviors of theirs make you angry. Avoid saying things like, "You make me mad," or "It's your fault." Appeal to their good nature and keep conversations light but insightful.

It's also crucial that you learn to explain to others how you feel. Say things like, "I'm really sorry, but I feel kind of anxious right now. It's making me feel a little agitated and angry. I think this is more about me than you, so let me deal with it a little bit." Ask for space to breathe for a moment if you need to. Avoid developing a behavioral pattern where your first response to an angry trigger is to react.

You might find that you become angry when your children disagree with you. Instead of getting mad at them, take a breath. Then ask them why they disagree and try to find a middle ground. This will also teach them valuable negotiation and communication skills they can use throughout their lives.

If you are a parent to a teenager, you might feel ignored or abandoned when your children choose to spend time and energy on their peer group and external friendships rather than with you and the family. This could express itself as an angry response when your children say they would rather do something with their friends than attend a celebratory dinner to mark a special family occasion. Talk to them about your feelings, explaining that you want them to participate in this event, as you would like to share it with them.

Keep an anger journal. Write down your experiences with anger as a way to reflect and understand what is happening. This is often encouraged by psychotherapists as a means to express anger and darker thoughts without harming others. Many people find that writing down how they feel helps them relieve the pressure of their feelings without affecting the people around them.

COMMUNICATE WITH YOUR CHILDREN

Effective communication is critical for good parent-child relationships. It's about listening to their side of the story and seeing things from their perspective. This is also the time to apologize, especially if you had a particularly ugly, angry outburst. You may have shown a violent face to your child. It is time to take responsibility for your behavior.

One of the issues plaguing society today is that people don't listen to one another—and the same goes for parents. Make a concerted effort to truly listen to your children and give them your attention when they speak to you, especially if they are angry. Be careful not to jump to conclusions too quickly. Children find it hard to control their anger, especially if their parents wrongly accuse them. If they are not allowed to express their feelings, this can ultimately lead to them having anger issues themselves when they are adults.

Active listening can also help. Not everything that's said by others needs to affect you. Let others say what they want to say. If they involve you, simply reflect back to them what they said to you without judging them.

Anger can come from the way in which someone is brought up. One man explained on social media: "My parents were very controlling, and I was never allowed to do much. Now, after 13 years of marriage, I find myself getting angry with my wife if I feel she is asking too many questions. I am angry when my kids make a mess or don't tidy up after themselves. I hate being criticized too."

Another said, "I was never allowed to express my opinion on anything. I was constantly shouted at and given hidings. I was told flat-out that I was wrong if my father disagreed with my opinion. Sometimes, he couldn't be bothered to listen to me, so he'd just shout at me to shut up. As an adult, I tend to bottle things up and explode in a vicious cycle. Growing up like that meant I didn't know how to express my feelings appropriately or communicate properly in most of my relationships with others. However, I have now discovered why this happens. Although I am actively working on myself to change the way I relate to others, I still struggle."

TAKE ACTION TO RESOLVE THE TRIGGERS

When you have figured out what triggers you, stay ahead of the game and be proactive. Whether your triggers are visible or invisible, take action to deal with them. Stay away from negative people and instead surround yourself with positive individuals.

If you have an emotional pain response from your own life, remind yourself of this when your own children act out or have a tough time. Do not lash out at them, as it's not constructive to do so. Instead, seek professional help to deal with painful memories from your past to mitigate your invisible triggers.

KEEP YOUR TRIGGER LIST UP TO DATE

Different things will trigger you at different times. If you have gone through a stressful period or experienced a life-changing event, such as a bereavement, divorce, or a house move, you might find yourself more likely to give into your anger at these times. Allow yourself time to feel the emotions such events bring and then let them go. Be kind to yourself. Take warm, candlelit baths, long walks, or have long conversations with good friends.

Foster awareness and update your list if you find that different things are triggering you. Be patient with yourself as you relearn your responses to experiences and events that trigger your angry emotions.

It's important not to be afraid of your emotions. Humans are emotional beings, and our feelings reveal not only who we are but what we are experiencing. They show us the things we really need, including fears that we should overcome, sadness that requires grieving, or anger that needs to be processed in a healthy way. It's not "wrong" to be angry, any more than it's "wrong" to be happy or sad. The issue is how you handle your anger (or not).

Anger is often unresolved frustration, and if the reasons for your frustration are not addressed, it can fester, often venting as a violent explosion. Work on addressing the reasons behind your anger rather than simply trying to rein it in. If you cannot justify your anger, you are less likely to break your anger habit. Here are a few helpful questions you can ask yourself:

- What is triggering my anger (why do I feel this way)?
- How could I express my feelings productively?
- Am I using my feelings as an excuse to mistreat others?
- Am I entitled to behave badly just because I feel angry?

You are not a robot. You are a human being, and every one of us has thoughts and emotions. Anyone who says they don't have any feelings is deceiving themselves.

Focus on your emotion and what triggered it. Did the person who sparked your anger actually mean well but misinterpret the situation? Did something happen? Would it help to shout at your children or hurt someone and regret it later? Wouldn't it be better to talk about the situation in a calm, rational way? If the trigger is a situation you can't resolve or an expectation that wasn't met, what can you do to change it? Will getting angry change it?

Evaluating the situation and deciding on an appropriate response will help you better deal with your angry feelings. You will become more empowered as you realize that you can choose how to resolve a situation rather than having a knee-jerk response based on negative thoughts, which can ultimately push people away.

USE CALMING HERBS

Herbal remedies have been used through the ages to address numerous common physical and mental ailments. Made into teas, fresh or dried herbs can help promote calmness and serenity. Several herbal essential oils can also relieve stress, anxiety, and frustration and promote calm after a shock, such as a bereavement or accident.

If any herb does not agree with you or results in skin rash, headaches, or other discomforts, discontinue use immediately. If you are on blood thinners or blood pressure medication, consult your health practitioner before using herbs, as many affect blood pressure or thin the blood.

Herbs for anxiety, stress, and the nervous system can be divided into nervines and adaptogens.

Nervines

Nervines are plants or herbs used to regulate and balance the nervous system. They are usually divided into relaxants, stimulants, and tonics.

- Tonics are used to aid recovery after exposure to extreme stress or trauma and for treating

addiction. Nervine tonics are known for their therapeutic properties and are particularly useful when taken over an extended period. The herbal compounds build up in the body while targeting nerve tissues.
- Nervine relaxants calm the nervous system, promoting serenity. They can be used anytime and are known to soothe the mind and digestive system.
- On the other side of the spectrum, nervine stimulants excite the nervous system, bringing mind and body into balance and harmony. They should not be used by those inclined to be anxious or excitable.

Nervines for Serenity

Chamomile has been used as a calmative since the 14th century (Roberts, 2012). Originally a European wildflower, it has been naturalized in North America. Besides anxiety and stress, it relieves stomach upsets and indigestion, and promotes sleep. To make the tea, add one teaspoon of fresh or dried flowers to one cup of boiling water. Strain after five minutes, and sip slowly (Roberts, 2012). The tea may be drunk hot or cold, or added to fruit juice to make a refreshing, calming drink.

Lavender is soothing and smells delicious. The essential oil is known for calming anxiety and reducing stress. Add three drops to the bathwater after the bath has run and relax in the fragrant steam (Roberts, 2012). Lavender also has pain-relieving and anti-inflammatory properties. You can also make tea from the flowers. Pour a cup of boiling water over a quarter of a cup of fresh or dried flowers, steep for five minutes, and sip slowly after discarding the plant material (Roberts, 2012).

Valerian has been used since the 2nd century for anxiety, nervous restlessness, and as a sleep aid (Mount Sinai, n.d.). In Germany, it was approved for use as a mild sedative. It is believed that it works by increasing the amount of gamma-aminobutyric acid (GABA) in the brain. This helps regulate the nerve cells and calms anxiety. It is believed to produce a similar effect to drugs such as Xanax and Valium. The effect of valerian increases over time and may be combined with hops and lemon balm to treat insomnia. The root is usually used, made into a powder or tincture. Valerian may interact with other sedatives, antihistamines, statins, or alcohol, so check with your healthcare practitioner before using valerian.

Hops are better known as the primary ingredient in beer, but did you know that the flowers have long been used for irritability, sleeplessness, and various digestive ailments? An herbal tea made from flowers helps to relieve exhaustion and stress. To make the tea, pour a cup of boiling water over a quarter of a cup of fresh leaves, let the tea steep for five minutes, then strain and sip slowly. If you wish to use the tea for insomnia, take one cup twice daily. Drink the second cup at bedtime (Roberts, 2015).

California poppies, originally used as a painkiller and a sedative, have today become a valuable "rescue remedy." Compounds in the plant promote a gentle calmness that brings relief from stress. Harvest this Californian wildflower in full bloom and dry the petals for quick relief. It is safe for both young and old to use. The plant is used to relieve insomnia, hyperactivity, over-excitement, and over-stimulation—and it's antispasmodic to boot. It can also be given to children with behavioral problems.

Adaptogens

These herbs and plants help ease the body's natural response to stress. Adaptogenic plants need to be non-toxic and safe, enabling the body to combat stress and rebalance it. Adaptogens help to regulate the production of stress hormones and manage the body's "fight-or-flight" response.

Adaptogenic Herbs

Ashwagandha boosts the immune system and is excellent for relieving long-term stress. It has a neuroprotective action, is a safe sedative, and is also used as a tonic. It should not be used if you are on sleeping pills or pregnant, as it stimulates the uterus.

Rosavin, also known as rhodiola, is known for its stress- and fatigue-reducing properties. It also enables clear thinking, especially when under pressure. It alleviates psychological stress and anxiety in particular and is believed to moderate the release of cortisol when stress is experienced.

Saffron is a rare but valuable spice that is sometimes referred to as the "sunshine spice." It is known for its ability to cheer you up and relieve dark moods. It is ideal for combating anger, anxiety, and depression. Over-the-counter saffron extracts improve concentration and alleviate irritation naturally.

Lemon balm, a plant that belongs to the mint family, helps to promote sleep, relieve pain, and reduce anxiety and stress. It can also help to combat depression. Make the fresh herb into a refreshing, calming tea. It has a pleasant lemony taste.

If you thought turmeric was only good for curries, think again. Curcumin, which gives the root its yellow pigment, is an excellent anti-inflammatory. Better known as a circulatory spice, turmeric is traditionally used in India for anxiety. Add a teaspoon of turmeric powder to a little hot water and drink it for quick relief (Roberts, 2012).

OTHER USEFUL SUPPLEMENTS FOR ANGER MANAGEMENT

Are you getting enough vitamin B? Vitamin B is known for feeding the nerves and is typically found in foods such as grains, oily fish, and eggs. Vitamin B complex supplements usually contain several different B vitamins. Ingesting adequate quantities of vitamin B will lift your mood, reduce stress, and raise your energy levels. People who take vitamin B supplements get angry less often and are less fatigued and stressed.

Melatonin is another valuable supplement for combating anger. It's typically associated with better sleep (your body produces melatonin when it starts getting dark, preparing you for sleep), but it also reduces anxiety and aggression.

L-theanine is an amino acid produced by tea leaves, which is often included in supplements used for anger relief. The extract both increases alertness and has a calming effect without causing drowsiness. It also decreases the physical effects of anger, reducing the heart rate.

An amino acid called 5-hydroxytryptophan (5-HTP) is often included in sleeping and anti-anxiety supplements. It is converted to serotonin in the body, which lifts the mood while reducing stress. It also calms those angry feelings and promotes better sleep.

7

THREE KEY INGREDIENTS TO RAISE WILLING, SELF-REGULATED CHILDREN

> *The most precious inheritance that parents can give their children is their own happiness.*
>
> — THICH NHAT HANH

In this chapter, you will discover the three principles of raising willing, self-regulated children: Building a relationship, having open communication, expressing emotions in an open, healthy way, and loving unconditionally.

FOSTERING A GOOD RELATIONSHIP

The most important thing for a parent is to develop a relationship with their children that creates a strong, real, and lasting bond. They may be your children today, but one day they will be adults and will be forming their own relationships. If you build a good relationship with them, this will show them how to develop sound ones with other people later in life.

Connect with Your Child

As a parent, it's extremely important to sit down with your children, give them your complete attention, and ask them about their day. Have a time of day when you all put your phones away—or on silent—keep the television off and spend quality time with one another. This can also be done at mealtimes. Rather than having a TV dinner, eat supper at the table and talk to one another about your days.

Another thing parents can do for and with their children is to do sporting and other physical activities with them, so exercise becomes a routine but enjoyable experience. This encourages children to develop healthy lifestyles. Get them to shop and cook with you and teach them about healthy eating. Make their health and safety your top priority.

Even if you're a busy parent, make an effort to spend the free time you have with them intentionally. Play, cuddle, and laugh freely. Read to them—or let them read to you. Share stories about the family, go for walks, or enjoy urban adventures together. The more time you spend with them, especially when they're young, the better the foundation you will build as they get older.

Today, too many parents seem to ignore their children. After spending time on necessary errands and chores after a workday, parents focus on some entertainment to unwind rather than taking time out to be with their children. Some parents may also find their children "boring" and would rather interact with adults or work colleagues. This means that many children grow up feeling neglected on some level. They may have everything they need or want materially—except their parent's time and attention, which is what they need and desire most of all.

Our culture tends to foster this: Parenting advice suggests that we should allow children to cry because it's not the right time to feed them, or because they should get used to sleeping alone or to encourage a sleeping routine that gives parents a break.

The real—and often hidden—power of parenting is when your children genuinely want to belong to you and have a relationship with you. They are interested in maintaining it on their end as well. Unless there is a relationship between the two of you, a child won't want to be with you.

If you have not built a proper relationship with your child, you are more likely to have conflicts when you want to offer your children guidance or set boundaries. This is one of the key reasons why children, especially when they are teenagers, rebel against their parents.

The Dutch raise their children very differently from the way Americans do. While American parents tend to expose their children to countless new experiences all the time, Dutch parents focus on day-to-day activities and chores at home. They place a lot of emphasis on having a proper routine and everyone in the family getting enough rest.

In 1996, the Dutch government gave part-time workers the same rights as full-time ones, allowing more flexibility in the workplace to foster a better work-life balance. This has resulted in nearly half the population working part-time, regardless of their work and profession. Many Dutch men work just four days a week, allowing them to spend an entire day with their children (Acosta, 2019). This has become so much the norm that the Dutch call it "papadag" or "father's day." Unsurprisingly, Dutch children are considered among the happiest in the world!

Today, parenting is often regarded as a role one plays, but it's actually about developing a relationship with your children—no more and no less. This isn't something that comes with no strings attached. It takes time, attention, and effort. You can't transfer it from another relationship, like when you become a step-parent due to the child's mother marrying you after a divorce or a bereavement.

Creating a Nourishing, Non-Toxic Environment

One of the parents' primary tasks is to ensure that they provide a nourishing, safe environment where their children can grow up. It's essential to give children help and support in becoming the people they will one day be. Avoid imposing unrealistic expectations on your children regarding whom they will become or what professions they will pursue after school.

I was not good at ELA when I was at school—it simply wasn't my forte—but I was an A-grade student in math. One end-of-term, I brought home a report card where I had barely passed ELA and was concerned about what my father would say. When he got home, he duly looked at our report cards. I apologized for my low ELA grades. He asked me, "Did you do your best?" Surprised, I told him that I had. He then said, "We know that you are not great at English. If this is your best, then it's good enough. But if you got this grade for math, then I would be upset because we all know your math is excellent." I realized then that the most important thing was to give everything my best shot, even if I wasn't very good at it.

There are no "good" or "bad" children, although some will be happier and some will be kinder. If parents create a caring environment that doesn't pressure their children to be something they are not, they will tend to behave better. However, if you continually yell and shout, children will misbehave and may even become downright nasty.

If your children also have anger issues, being in a toxic family environment can be very detrimental, fostering their frustration and encouraging them to suppress their feelings and later explode. Suppose children grow up in situations where there is constant bickering, yelling and shouting, sarcasm, spite, recrimination, or even verbal or physical abuse. In that case, this can create invisible triggers for childhood anger that spills over into adulthood. It can also lead to other mental health issues.

One teen commented on social media, "Whenever my mom opens her mouth, I just want to throw something. It's not what she says. I remember all the times she hurt me, and I went into flight mode." As a child, if your relationship with one of your parents was toxic, you might have found that nothing you did was good enough. Their relationship with you was always on their terms, and they were never accountable for their actions. Toddlers, for example, may not always understand the words you use, but they certainly appreciate the volume and the tone of your voice.

ALLOW FREEDOM OF EXPRESSION

It's important to allow your children to express their emotions within reason and with parental guidance. They need to learn to talk about their feelings and struggles instead of holding them inside themselves.

This can even be done when your children are small. If your toddler refuses to hold your hand when you need to cross a busy road on foot, take him aside, bend down to his level, and talk to him: "I know you don't want to do this, but you need to do this to be safe. You can let go of my hand when we get to the park."

Tell your children that it is okay for them to experience emotions, whether they are angry, sad, confused, embarrassed, or whatever it is. Empathize with them and show them how to deal with it. Talk to them about the events that made them feel that way and suggest to them how they can defuse their emotions. Discuss how they might deal with that difficult teacher, the girl in their class who is bullying them, or the boy they don't like who keeps pestering them. Very often, children get angry because they are not being heard.

This happens from early childhood: No one listens to young children because they are small. They are simply expected to do what they are told, as though they aren't real people. Parents need to make time for their children while they are young, which engenders trust. If you explode every time your child approaches you about something small, they will have no reason to talk to you about bigger things. A lot of parents' emotions are triggered by those of their children. They themselves may have been bottling up their feelings for years in the interests of pleasing others or fitting in socially. This means they don't really know how to process their own feelings, let alone those of others.

Never discourage a child from expressing their emotions. They have every right to have feelings and need to be taught how to manage them positively. When children own their feelings, they also learn how to express them appropriately. This teaches them self-discipline and how to think for themselves. When parents yell or shout, their children tend to shut down simply because the parents' fury is much more significant.

Remember that listening is probably the best thing you can do for your children. Today, many of us listen only to reply. But listening—and paying attention to their interactions—is an excellent way to see the world from your children's perspective. Your children know when you're listening actively and they're being heard—and they will know that they are valuable in your eyes. Validate their feelings—and remember to be open about yours, too, so they learn how to express emotions in a positive way. Face conflicts head-on, together, so they don't get a chance to blow up out of proportion or to fester.

Recognize that you are not a perfect parent. There will be times when you express your anger and scream or shout at your children. Once the storm is over, it's important to climb down, apologize to your children, explain what went wrong, and discuss how to handle the situation in the future. Sometimes the problem is simply a miscommunication or a misunderstanding, but this can affect a relationship negatively if it is allowed to linger.

You could also have regular family meetings, so your children feel they are part of a team working towards common goals. Allow your children to voice their opinions. Even if you and your spouse will ultimately make the decisions, your children will feel valued and appreciated. Explain how doing chores enables them to contribute to the family and the home. Eat together as a family as often as possible. This can be invaluable for building family relationships.

It was an unwritten rule in our house that we all sat down at the dining room table nearly every night. The television and radio were switched off. We'd put aside our books and newspapers, homework, sewing, or whatever other projects we were all doing. We'd talk about our days over dinner—things we had done, people we knew, or things that had been on the news. Often, a discussion would continue after the meal was over—and we'd sit for hours talking over mugs of coffee until we exhausted the subject.

Teaching your children to be assertive from an early age is also important. In Dutch families, everyone has a say. This means that, from a relatively early age, children are able to set boundaries as to what they are comfortable with or things they don't like or want. Everything effectively becomes a negotiation. This type of parenting is demanding work, but it will teach your child a skill that can be invaluable later in life. As a parent, you need to make it clear that there are rules and that you also have boundaries because of that: Your children cannot do or have everything they want, as not everything is beneficial for them. For instance, a young child needs to go to bed at a particular time so they won't be tired the next day. It would not be suitable for them to play with a sharp knife or scissors, as they could hurt themselves. Explain to your child why you are setting these rules so that they learn to understand that you are not being unreasonable but are protecting them.

Being assertive is often characterized by being direct and to the point. The habit of assertiveness—being direct in a respectful way—means you don't get annoyed because you can clearly state your needs. Americans often criticize Dutch people for being too direct, even to the point of bluntness. They tend to say what they mean. On the plus side, they are more likely to be calm and rarely lose their tempers. Dutch culture allows people to have an opinion and to express themselves assertively. In fact, lack of assertiveness is considered a health problem and was even covered by health insurance in the past!

LOVING UNCONDITIONALLY

George Valliant, who directed a 30-year Harvard Grant Study focusing on personal happiness, concluded that those who are the most satisfied with their lives are highly likely to have had several warm, close relationships throughout their lifetimes.

Happiness Engenders Success

Albert Schweitzer said, "Success is not the key to happiness. Happiness is the key to success. If you love what you are doing, you will be successful." (BrainyQuote, n.d.).

Neurological studies of positive psychology prove that happiness is a crucial driver and precursor of success. This is because positive feelings make the brain work better.

Dutch parents—like all parents—have lofty ambitions for their children. In their culture, happiness is generally regarded as a path to success rather than the other way around. Happiness also enhances self-awareness, motivates, creates independence, and encourages people to develop strong ties with their communities. This all helps to create success.

It's essential to allow children to do things they enjoy rather than forcing them to be what you want them to be. Respect your children's goals, dreams, beliefs, privacy, preferences, friends, etc. Never joke about or mock their choices. This is especially important for teens. If they are loved, they will be less likely to rebel when they reach this life stage.

Never giving your children any privacy will only make them anxious or resentful. If you check your children's phones every night, they will become concerned, even if they have nothing to hide.

It's also important to have an open dialogue with your children. It is obvious that there needs to be a level of respect on their part. Still, there is nothing like your teenager feeling comfortable enough with you to ask your opinions and have discussions about just about anything. They will ultimately develop their own tastes and opinions, which means you need to give them some leeway while still keeping them in check and being there to support them.

Every morning when you wake up, tell yourself: Today, I will give my children the best gift—my own happiness.

HELP ANOTHER PARENT WITH JUST ONE CLICK

As you begin to embrace a calmer outlook, you may wish you'd come across this information sooner. You may not be able to go back in time, but you can help make the road a little easier for someone else.

Simply by sharing your honest opinion of this book on Amazon, you'll show new readers where they can find the guidance they need to manage their anger.

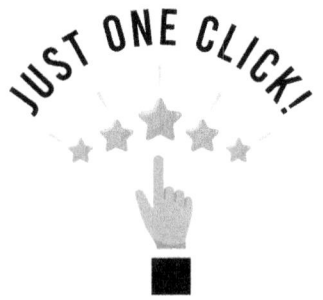

Thank you so much for your support. Our anger hurts us just as much as it hurts our children… It's my mission to reduce that pain.

Scan the QR code for a quick review!

CONCLUSION

Anger is real—and it's a powerful emotion. When you are ready to erupt like a volcano, your feelings can take over your mind and body, and it can be hard to keep a cool head. Anger feeds on itself, so the more often you give vent to it and become angry, the angrier you will be overall. Angry parents also beget angry children: They learn these negative, destructive behaviors from infancy and grow up irritable, prone to fits of fury and tunnel vision rage.

But it doesn't have to be this way. Anger is the tip of the emotional iceberg, and it's a secondary emotion because we almost always feel something else before we get angry, like fear, sadness, or disgust. Sometimes, society has taught us not to express such feelings, so they are masked by anger.

Our upbringing could predispose us to anger if our parents constantly criticized us, falsely accused us of doing wrong, ignored us, or compared us endlessly with our siblings, for instance. People who experience this sort of behavior as children may suffer from reduced feelings of self-worth or even depression, which manifests in explosive outbursts.

Exploding is a negative way of expressing anger, as it inevitably leads to more of the same—and people who get angry like this often find themselves sucked into a vicious cycle that they seem unable to break free of. It also frightens those around them and drives people away. In extreme cases, anger can turn into aggression, leading to physical violence and trouble with the law.

Biologically, anger is part of the body's fight-or-flight response, which kicks in when we experience real or perceived threats. This releases hormones such as adrenaline and cortisol, enabling us to defend ourselves physically. But, if anger dominates your personality, being constantly in a state of anger and stress can have a slew of adverse health impacts. In extreme cases, anger can cause life-threatening health issues—and it can literally end up killing you over time.

As parents, we need to guard ourselves against expressing our anger in a knee-jerk fashion. After all, we don't want to raise angry, antisocial people. The first step in bringing your rage under control—particularly if it has a destructive impact on your home and family—is to identify your triggers. These can be visible, as in situations that make you angry, or invisible, as in past events that manifest as anger in the present.

If invisible triggers cause your anger, addressing the emotions and underlying issues behind your anger is essential. Get professional help if necessary. The positive outcome is that your anger will be an annoyance; it won't be clouded and compounded by past events.

There are various techniques one can use to diffuse anger. Exercising, taking a breath, thinking positive thoughts, taking a bath, or washing your face are ways to prevent anger from taking over and ruling you in a given situation. You can also use a 3-step method developed by ancient Taoist practitioners to provide quick relief and enable you to function without going off the deep end at every opportunity.

Practice mindfulness to become aware of your triggers and know when they are in play. Anger *is* manageable and controllable. If you take the time to pay attention and address your anger issues, you will ultimately see progress. However, you need to be patient with yourself: Rome wasn't built in a day, and managing your anger will take time. You will need to practice mitigation skills even when you're not angry. Practice makes perfect, and mindfulness is ultimately the key to preventing your angry emotions from getting the upper hand.

It's important to build a good relationship with your children, considering their point of view, setting appropriate boundaries, and understanding their development and changing needs at different stages of their lives. When you control your anger and express your requirements and needs in a calm, constructive manner, you, in turn, teach them to manage their own emotions when they feel irritable or annoyed. This builds serene adults who can make their way in the adult world without being triggered by its demands or when things don't work out the way they planned.

Anger is a powerful emotion, and it's vital to ensure that we can manage and control it rather than letting it control us. I hope this book will help you begin your journey to calmness and wholeness so that anger is no longer a destructive force but a constructive experience.

REFERENCES

Achieve Medical Center. (2020, November 29). *Your brain thrives on positivity*. Achieve Medical Center. https://www.achievemedicalcenter.com/blog-post/your-brain-thrives-on-positivity#rmation:~:

Acosta, R. M. (2019, June 6). *I spent 7 years studying Dutch parenting—here are 6 secrets to raising the happiest kids in the world*. CNBC. https://www.cnbc.com/2019/06/06/dutch-parenting-secrets-to-raising-the-happiest-kids-in-the-world.html.html

Advocate Arora Health. (2013, September 6). *Yelling at teens may just reinforce bad behavior*. Health Enews. https://www.aurorahealthcareblog.org/2013/09/06/yelling-at-teens-may-just-reinforce-bad-behavior/

American Psychological Association. (n.d.). *Anger and aggression*. https://www.apa.org/topics/anger

Amritha K. (2021, July 9). *Anger foods 101: Foods that can cause anger, such as tomato, brinjal, and foods that help manage anger*. https://www.boldsky.com. https://www.boldsky.com/health/wellness/anger-foods-list-of-foods-that-can-cause-anger-and-foods-that-help-manage-anger-137698.html

Be Herbal. (2020, October 28). *Effective therapies and herbal supplements for anger management*. Be Herbal®. https://www.beherbal.com/blogs/post/supplements-for-anger

Bhandi, S. (2022, August 25). *Why am I so angry?* WebMD. https://www.webmd.com/balance/guide/why-am-i-so-angry

Bible Study Tools. (2021, March 30). *Anger Bible verses*. Biblestudytools.com. https://www.biblestudytools.com/topical-verses/anger-bible-verses/

Brainy Quote. (n.d.). *Top 10 anger quotes*. BrainyQuote. Retrieved December 4, 2022, from https://www.brainyquote.com/lists/topics/top-10-anger-quotes

BrainyQuote. (n.d.). *Albert Schweitzer quotes.* BrainyQuote. https://www.brainyquote.com/quotes/albert_schweitzer_155988

Brooks, L. (2010). *The differences between catecholamines and cortisol. Sciencing.* https://sciencing.com/differences-between-catecholamines-cortisol-7472976.html

Brullis, J. (2020, April 27). *Is watching the news making your anxiety worse? Tips for staying informed and managing anxiety.* Adaa.org. https://adaa.org/learn-from-us/from-the-experts/blog-posts/consumer/watching-news-making-your-anxiety-worse-tips

Burkhardt, M. (2020, January 9). *You are not what you think you are—The false self, the ego, and the true self.* Ascent Publication. https://medium.com/the-ascent/you-are-not-what-you-think-you-are-the-false-self-the-ego-and-the-true-self-13064f51918e

Center for Clinical Psychology. (n.d.). *Basic emotions.* Centre for Clinical Psychology Melbourne. https://ccp.net.au/basic-emotions/

Center for Disease Control and Prevention. (2021, February 22). *Adolescence (15-17 years old).* Centers for Disease Control and Prevention. https://www.cdc.gov/ncbddd/childdevelopment/positiveparenting/adolescence2.html

Centers for Disease Control and Prevention. (2019). *Young teens (12-14 years old).* Centers for Disease Control and Prevention. https://www.cdc.gov/ncbddd/childdevelopment/positiveparenting/adolescence.html

Child Mind Institute. (n.d.). *Angry kids: Dealing with explosive behavior.* Child Mind Institute. Retrieved December 2, 2022, from https://childmind.org/article/angry-kids-dealing-with-explosive-behavior/#top_of_page

Cleveland Clinic. (2022, May 19). *Endorphins: What they are and how to boost them.* Cleveland Clinic. https://my.clevelandclinic.org/health/body/23040-endorphins Colvin, M. (2022, February 18). *Understanding (and taming) your COVID anger.* www.wbur.org. https://www.wbur.org/cognoscenti/2022/02/18/pandemic-fatigue-anger-anxiety-molly-colvin

Cutler, N. (2011, October 13). *Anger inflames liver disease.* LiverSupport.com. https://www.liversupport.com/anger-inflames-

REFERENCES | 175

liver-disease/

Daube, PhD, E. (n.d.). *Where does anger stem from?* www.quora.com. Retrieved November 12, 2022, from https://www.quora.com/search?q=fast%20track%20message%20is%20sent%20to%20the%20amygdala%20&type=answer

Direction Psychology. (n.d.). *The importance of me time.* Direction Psychology. https://www.directionpsychology.com/article/the-importance-of-me-time/

Dougherty, E. (2022). *Anger management.* Hms.harvard.edu. https://hms.harvard.edu/magazine/science-emotion/anger-management

Dr. Christian Conte. (2016). *5 keys to controlling anger.* On YouTube. https://www.youtube.com/watch?v=KH3PHGjpo5Y

Dyslin, A. (2022, June 15). *Does the pandemic have you "pangry"?* Mayo Clinic News Network. https://newsnetwork.mayoclinic.org/discussion/does-the-pandemic-have-you-pangry/

Frank, K., Patel, K., Lopez, G., & Willis, B. (2021). *Rhodiola rosea research analysis.* Examine.com. https://examine.com/supplements/rhodiola-rosea/

Gerrie, H. (2020, June 10). *Our second brain: More than a gut feeling.* UBC Neuroscience. https://neuroscience.ubc.ca/our-second-brain-more-than-a-gut-feeling/

Gold, G. (2013, November 12). *How your moods mess with your skin.* EverydayHealth.com. https://www.everydayhealth.com/beauty-pictures/how-moods-mess-with-your-skin.aspx

Green, A. (2017, September 26). *Psychological development in puberty.* How to Adult. https://howtoadult.com/psychological-development-puberty-5337.html

Gupta, A. (2021, November 26). *Stress aside, these 3 emotions can impact your gut health.* Healthshots. https://www.healthshots.com/mind/emotional-health/gut-brain-connection-stress-can-affect-your-gut-health/

Hanson, R. (2011, September 26). *How to trick your brain for happiness.* Greater Good. https://greatergood.berkeley.edu/article/item/how_to_trick_your_brain_for_happiness

Health Direct. (2019, February 20). *Exercise and mental health.*

Healthdirect.gov.au; Healthdirect Australia. https://www.healthdirect.gov.au/exercise-and-mental-health

Involved Staff. (2021, November 14). *Put yourself in your kid's shoes to become a better parent.* www.involvedk12.org. https://www.involvedk12.org/resources/put-yourself-in-a-kids-shoes-to-become-a-better-parent

Jain, S. (2017, June 1). *5 tips to improve digestion.* www.practo.com. https://www.practo.com/healthfeed/5-tips-to-improve-digestion-28490/post

Kabat-Zinn, J., & Hor, Tuck Loon (2007). *Arriving at your door: 108 lessons in mindfulness.* Hyperion.

Kassinove, H. (2021). *How to recognize and deal with anger.* Apa.org. https://www.apa.org/topics/anger/recognize

King, M. (2020, March 10). *10 ways to make yourself happy* - Homes For Students. Wearehomesforstudents.com. https://wearehomesforstudents.com/blog/health-and-wellbeing/simple-ways-to-make-yourself-happy

Kopperman, M. H. (n.d.). *Acupuncture: An overview of scientific evidence.* Evidence-Based Acupuncture. Retrieved November 23, 2022, from https://www.evidencebasedacupuncture.org/acupuncture-scientific-evidence/#:~:text=Research%20into%20acupuncture

Kubzansky, L. D., Sparrow, D., Jackson, B., Cohen, S., Weiss, S. T., & Wright, R. J. (2006). *Angry breathing: A prospective study of hostility and lung function in the normative aging study.* Thorax, 61(10), 863–868. https://doi.org/10.1136/thx.2005.050971

Larsen, D. A. (2016, May 1). *Acupuncture point: Conception vessel 17 (CV 17).* Acupuncture Technology News. https://www.miridiatech.com/news/2016/05/acupuncture-point-conception-vessel-17/

Leinwand, L. (2016, November 10). *Why is saying "no" so important?* GoodTherapy.org Therapy Blog. https://www.goodtherapy.org/blog/why-is-saying-no-so-important-1110165 Lewis, A. (2021, May 26). *Ren 17.* Mend Acupuncture. https://mendacupuncture.com/ren-17/

Liang, F., & Wu, X. (2006). *The developmental status and prospect of the science of acupuncture and moxibustion abroad.* Zhongguo Zhen Jiu =

Chinese Acupuncture & Moxibustion, 26(2). https://pubmed.ncbi.nlm.nih.gov/16541850/

Live On Purpose TV. (2017). *How to get kids to listen without yelling.* On YouTube. https://www.youtube.com/watch?v=kHvm1J9HVLo

Lively, S. (2015, May 31). *What you need to know about parenting triggers.* One Time Through. https://onetimethrough.com/what-you-need-to-know-about-parenting-triggers/

Loewenberg, A. (2019). *When it comes to infant-toddler care and development, it's all about the relationships.* New America. https://www.newamerica.org/education-policy/edcentral/when-it-comes-infant-toddler-care-and-development-its-all-about-relationships/

Lyall, S. (2022, January 14). *Why is everyone so angry? We investigated.* The New York Times. https://www.nytimes.com/2022/01/14/insider/why-is-everyone-so-angry-we-investigated.html

Maitre, P. (n.d.). *When is it good to be angry?* Quora. Retrieved November 12, 2022, from https://www.quora.com/When-is-it-good-to-be-angry

Maoshing Ni. (1995). *The yellow emperor's classic of medicine: A new translation of the Neijing Suwen with Commentary.* Shambhala.

Miholic, I. I. (2018). *How do you minimize sibling rivalry?* Quora. https://www.quora.com/How-do-you-minimize-sibling-rivalry?q=How%20to%20minimize%20sibling%20rivalry%20for%20parents

Mind. (2017). *About anxiety.* www.mind.org.uk. https://www.mind.org.uk/information-support/types-of-mental-health-problems/anxiety-and-panic-attacks/about-anxiety/

Moeller, H.-G. . (2012). *Taoism.* Encyclopedia of Applied Ethics, 298–305. https://doi.org/10.1016/b978-0-12-373932-2.00217-9

Motivation Thrive. (2020). *How to become a better parent: Positive vs. toxic parenting tips. Dr. Gabor Maté.* On YouTube. https://www.youtube.com/watch?v=fcPPDbvGr7sgry/

Pittman, P. (2015, January 7). *Anger: A powerful emotion that can produce positive or negative results.* Alzheimer's Arkansas. https://www.alzark.org/anger-a-powerful-emotion-that-can-produce-positive-or-negative-results/#:~:text=Why%3F

Motivation Thrive. (2021). *How to control your anger | Jordan Peterson*

Life Advice. On YouTube. https://www.youtube.com/watch?v=hPoYX5FPtak

Mount Sinai. (n.d.). *Valerian information | Mount Sinai - New York.* Mount Sinai Health System. https://www.mountsinai.org/health-library/herb/valerian

New Hope Ranch. (2021, April 2). *Anger as a secondary emotion.* New Hope Ranch. https://www.newhoperanch.com/blog/understanding-anger-as-a-secondary-emotion/

Peterson, T. J. (2021, October 8). *Meditation for anger: How it works & tips for getting started.* Choosing Therapy. https://www.choosingtherapy.com/meditation-for-anger/

Pincus, D. (n.d.). *How to control your anger with kids.* Empowering Parents. https://www.empoweringparents.com/article/calm-parenting-get-control-child-making-an

Positive Parenting Solutions. (2009). *Sibling rivalry—positive parenting solutions.* Positive Parenting Solutions. https://www.positiveparentingsolutions.com/sibling-rivalry

Repanich, J. (2016, December 22). *This guy tried taking a deep breath every time he got pissed off. Here's what happened.* Men's Health. https://www.menshealth.com/health/a19534812/deep-breaths-when-angry/

Roberts, M. (2012). *My 100 favorite herbs.* Struik Nature.

Roberts, M., & Roberts, S. (2015). *100 New herbs.* Struik Nature.

Rozanski, A., Blumenthal, J. A., & Kaplan, J. (1999). Impact of psychological factors on the pathogenesis of cardiovascular disease and implications for therapy. Circulation, 99(16), 2192–2217. https://doi.org/10.1161/01.cir.99.16.2192

Sadhguru. (2018, October 27). *Sadhguru on how to never get angry or bothered by people.* www.youtube.com. https://www.youtube.com/watch?v=cxoQdEhHaT8

Schwartz, J. A., & Portnoy, J. (2017). Lower catecholamine activity is associated with greater levels of anger in adults. International Journal of Psychophysiology, 120(120), 33–41. https://doi.org/10.1016/j.ijpsycho.2017.07.005

Siegel, D., & Hartzell, M. (2005). *Parenting from inside out.* Thorsons.

Smarter Parenting. (2018). *How to control anger | Temper control for parents*. On www.youtube.com. https://www.youtube.com/watch?v=aYXEeaSSc7c

Soderlund, A. (n.d.). *Time-out vs. time-in: Is there a better way? Why you need the flexibility of a feeling break*. Nurture and Thrive. https://nurtureandthriveblog.com/feeling-break-time-in/

Soderlund, A. (2015, April 11). *What children teach us about life*. Nurture and Thrive. https://nurtureandthriveblog.com/what-children-teach-us-about-life/

Sources of Strength. (n.d.). *Breathing exercises*. Sources of Strength. https://sourcesofstrength.org/wp-content/uploads/Breathing.pdf

Summer, J. (2022, April 14). *Eight health benefits of sleep*. Sleep Foundation. https://www.sleepfoundation.org/how-sleep-works/benefits-of-sleep

Sutton, J. (2020, August 5). *Erik Erikson's stages of psychosocial development explained*. Positive Psychology. https://positivepsychology.com/erikson-stages/

Tengyuen, N. (2022, March 18). *41 quotes on anger management, controlling anger, and relieving stress*. GeckoandFly. https://www.geckoandfly.com/27904/anger-management-stress-quotes/

Veny, M. (2019, February 28). *Anger management: How to control anger. (Actionable!)*. www.youtube.com. https://www.youtube.com/watch?v=rUxbiqfNu8w

Westbrook, T. D. (2020, May 19). *Why is COVID-19 making me so angry?* Wexnermedical.osu.edu. https://wexnermedical.osu.edu/blog/why-so-angry-covid

Western Australia Department of Health. (2019, May 21). *Child development 0–3 months*. www.healthywa.wa.gov.au. https://www.healthywa.wa.gov.au/Articles/A_E/Child-development-0-3-months

Whole Family Happiness. (2018, March 2). *5 basics for building strong relationships with your kids*. The Whole Family Happiness Project. https://medium.com/the-whole-family-happiness-project/5-basics-for-building-strong-relationships-with-your-kids-fcaf7ccca3cb

Wikipedia. (2022, November 19). *Taoism*. Wikipedia. https://en.wikipedia.org/wiki/Taoism

Wikipedia Contributors. (2018, June 10). *Grant study*. Wikipedia; Wikimedia Foundation. https://en.wikipedia.org/wiki/Grant_Study

Wikipedia Contributors. (2019, October 21). *The 100: A ranking of the most influential persons in history*. Wikipedia; Wikimedia Foundation. https://en.wikipedia.org/wiki/The_100:_A_Ranking_of_the_Most_Influential_Persons_in_History

WishGarden Herbs. (2022, August 13). *What the hell are nervines, adaptogens and alteratives?* – WishGarden Herbs. www.wishgardenherbs.com. https://www.wishgardenherbs.com/blogs/wishgarden/what-are-nervines-adaptogens-and-alteratives

Zugaro, M. (2022, September 8). *I stopped watching news 6 years ago—here's why you should quit, too*. Age of Awareness. https://medium.com/age-of-awareness/i-stopped-watching-news-6-years-ago-heres-why-you-should-quit-too-225c66e102e2

IMAGE REFERENCES

Woodley, Sasha. 2022. *Anger iceberg*
Woodley, Sasha. 2022. *CV 17*

Printed in Great Britain
by Amazon